# The Successful Physician

## A Productivity Handbook for Practitioners

### Marshall O. Zaslove, MD

Director
The Zaslove Group
Napa, California

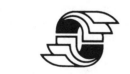

AN ASPEN PUBLICATION®
Aspen Publishers, Inc.
Gaithersburg, Maryland
1998

**Library of Congress Cataloging-in-Publication Data**

Zaslove, Marshall O.
The successful physician: a productivity handbook for
practitioners/Marshall O. Zaslove.
p. cm.
Includes bibliographical references and index.
ISBN 0-8342-1098-3 (pbk.)
1. Medicine—Practice—Cost effectiveness—Handbooks, manuals, etc.
2. Medical offices—Management—Cost effectiveness—Handbooks, manuals, etc.
3. Physicians—Labor productivity—Handbooks, manuals, etc. I. Title.
R728.Z37 1998
610´.68—dc21
98-4368
CIP

Orders: (800) 638-8437
Customer Service: (800) 234-1660

**About Aspen Publishers** • For more than 35 years, Aspen has been a leading professional publisher in a variety of disciplines. Aspen's vast information resources are available in both print and electronic formats. We are committed to providing the highest quality information available in the most appropriate format for our customers. Visit Aspen's Internet site for more information resources, directories, articles, and a searchable version of Aspen's full catalog, including the most recent publications: **http://www.aspenpub.com**
**Aspen Publishers, Inc.** • The hallmark of quality in publishing
Member of the worldwide Wolters Kluwer group.

Editorial Services: Brian MacDonald
Library of Congress Catalog Card Number: 98-4368
ISBN: 0-8342-1098-3

*Printed in the United States of America*

1  2  3  4  5

*To*
*Darshan Singh*
*(1921–1989)*

*Poet, Teacher, Friend to All*

# Table of Contents

# Acknowledgments

The ideas and information in this book originally came from hundreds of physicians, nurses, and others who have participated in Physician Productivity Seminars since 1993. Then, three busy practitioners made time in their schedules to spend dozens of hours with me patiently discussing and shaping the raw material: D.M. Beale, MD; Catherine Mason, MD; and Dennis B. Bealick, MD.

Others who made crucial contributions include: B. Fetesoff, MLS, medical librarian; D. Garfinkle, seminar coach; R. Gervais, motivational expert; L. Veloso, RN; W. Cooper, RN; P. Ayers, RN; B. Mitchell, LVN; R. Tedding, RN; D. Gardner, RN; K. Barney, PT; C. Fry, BCCP; S. Trejo; and D. Marshall—all of whom helped with the sections on working in teams. My residents and patients also contributed their helpful ideas and opinions.

Several physicians helped out with anecdotes, encouragement, and editorial input, including: E. Brennan, MD; L. Bausch, MD; J. Stanton, MD; N. Varshney, MD; D. Edell, MD; F. Lu, MD; R. Beller, MD; H. Fox, MD; J. Gruft, MD; S. Shefayee, MD; I. Weitz, MD; R. Pineda, MD; T. Cedro, MD; H-S Yeh, MD, et al. Dave Harbaugh provided the curmudgeonly cartoons.

My wife Nina lovingly and patiently helped with the work over several years from planning to publication. Our daughters Natasha and Mira provided legal advice and editing, respectively.

Sandy Cannon, my editor at Aspen, had the vision of this book from early on, and guided it safely to its destination. Helping her (and me) was the great Aspen team, especially Kalen Conerly, Jennifer Barnes Eliot, and Brian MacDonald.

To every one of you, my heartfelt *Thanks*.

# Part 1

# How Can Physicians Become More Productive?

"To each one of you, the practice of medicine will be very much as you make it...to one a worry, a care, a perpetual annoyance; to another, a daily joy and a life of as much happiness and usefulness as can well fall to the lot of man."

Sir William Osler [1](p.423)

# How This Book Will Help You

## In the ICU, It's Never Amateur Night

Have you ever been seriously ill or injured—so seriously that you thought you might die?

It's a funny question to ask physicians. But everything goes in cycles. We're doctors now, but inevitably the cycle will turn, and each of us will someday get our chance to be a patient.

I fell gravely ill a few years ago, and found myself fighting for my life in our local hospital. Let me tell you what that feels like; if you've ever been very sick, you can judge whether it rings true.

When you're lying in a hospital bed, wondering if you're going to live or die, your whole world shrinks. You lose all interest in what's going on in the Middle East, or in Washington, DC, or on Wall Street. You even forget about your income taxes (this is assuming you're very sick).

In fact, the world shrinks until it's just the size of that tiny clot, smaller than the tip of your pinkie, which is clogging your coronary artery and threatening to kill you with a heart attack. Or it shrinks to the diameter of that quarter-sized shadow on your chest film, which may be a malignancy that could take your life. Or, if you're a woman, your world becomes as small as that marble-sized lump in your breast, which may be a cancer that could eat you alive.

When you're that sick and scared, and you look to the foot of the bed and see your doctor, believe me, you utter a fervent prayer that he or she is the best trained, most experienced, and most capable professional available. Every patient wants their physician to be a first-class practitioner who has spent every day of his working life battling toe-to-toe with little clots, or lung shadows, or breast lumps, or whatever is killing or paining them.

In short, every patient wants their physician to be someone like…you.

But there is real danger today that our very best practitioners— the most able and ethical among us—will give up medicine. On a recent survey, one out of every two doctors said they have considered leaving our profession.[2] There's hard evidence from disability statistics that physicians and surgeons are already exiting our profession in record numbers, taking with them their priceless wisdom and experience.[3]

## Why Doctors Are Quitting

The reasons doctors are pulling out will sound familiar to every practitioner:

- ✦ too much work and too little time to do it—many physicians are now seeing 50% more patients than they did a few years ago,[4] and almost all of us are trying to see more patients in less time
- ✦ relentless shrinking of doctors' fees, pay, and bonuses (adjusted for inflation, physician incomes have been going down)[5]
- ✦ increased competition and decreased job security
- ✦ more risk of liability and less autonomous control over our practices and our futures

✦ information overload and staff undertraining
✦ anger, frustration, depression, and the like

Faced with constant hassles in a professional milieu that's getting more and more stressful and less and less rewarding, it's no surprise that so many able practitioners are hanging it up.

## Our Mission: To Keep You in Practice

Our mission with this book is to show you *how to make your professional life easier*—more efficient, more productive, more satisfying, and safer for you and your patients.

In these pages you'll find more than 140 practical suggestions for reducing the hassles, pressures, worries, inefficiencies, and risks in your professional life. After all, this is a book about professional productivity—and if physicians get so annoyed and angry that they quit, their productivity automatically goes to zero.

But if even one skilled, seasoned, dedicated practitioner reads this book, puts to use some of the suggestions it contains, and so decides to hang on a little longer at the practice of his or her skills, then we will have accomplished our mission.

Doctors who actually tried some of the ideas in this book found they could make real, measurable differences in their practices. Recently, an intensivist in the Midwest wrote me to say that by adopting just one suggestion from the productivity seminar, he was saving one hour daily. That's 250 hours extra every working year—the equivalent of a four-week paid vacation!

Does that sound attractive to you?

## This Book Is about Real Solutions to Your Problems

In the next 16 chapters, we'll cover in detail the problems that affect us all these days; you'll definitely recognize some of the particular annoyances that make your professional life less satisfying than you want it to be.

What you'll be discovering as you read this book are methods that successful practitioners all over North America have developed in order to deal with these challenges. No one can telepathically see what you do 10 or 12 hours a day in your practice, and then tell you how to change your methods for the better; and because everyone's practice is unique, there aren't many general rules (there are some, however, and we'll get to them). But we have collected for you in this book the techniques which other physicians are using to make their work lives more pleasant and productive.

Going in, we want to emphasize that these suggestions come from busy practitioners very much like you; this is a report from the front, not a lecture. Physicians—generalists and specialists of every stripe—generously shared their wisdom in questionnaires; interviews; phone calls, letters, and e-mail; and after seminars, in dozens of impassioned, face-to-face discussions around podiums in hotel conference rooms, late in the afternoon, long after the crowds had left.

## The Physician Productivity Seminars

The material in this book was originally presented as a series of seminars given to audiences of physicians and surgeons around the U.S. and Canada over the past four years. Inevitably, each seminar became a spontaneous flow of ideas among colleagues, in which I always learned at least as much as I taught, and I'm deeply indebted to the hundreds of seminar participants who made practical suggestions and criticisms. Physicians honor the tradition of giving knowledge freely to colleagues, and these men and women who generously shared their treasures of savvy and experience for other physicians' benefit are this book's heroes.

Besides interviewing physicians and surgeons, we talked with nurses, medical and OR technicians, pharmacists, physician assistants, and office managers. Where we could find relevant research in the literature, we weighed its applicability to real-world problems before including it. Our patients and our families also quite freely expressed their views—so don't be surprised to find in these pages some candid feedback about how we come across to them.

Hundreds of seminar participants (and physicians who heard from colleagues about the seminar, but couldn't attend) have requested us to work up the information in our seminars into a handbook they could read, study, and use at their convenience. The book you're holding is our response to their requests.

## What You Will Get from This Book

Movie theaters used to post a sign in their box office announcing "Students $2.50" (or some such reduced admission). A bargain-priced movie house in San Francisco called The Surf had a different sign in their box office: "We Are All Students."

Indeed we are all still students—each of us can learn something useful from every other physician, if we're willing to listen to our colleagues.

> Medicine is a science, but practicing is an art; we learn it from other practitioners.

Before a recent seminar in California one physician complained: "How can I be any more productive than I am now? All I do is see patients, all day long." Two hours into the seminar, he came to the podium and said, "I had no idea how much I could be doing to make things go quicker and easier…I just never thought deeply enough about most of this stuff." As you read this book, you also may be surprised to see how much you can improve your efficiency.

If you had the time, you could take a few hundred hours off from your practice and conduct your own research, surveys, and interviews with other practitioners to find out what they're doing to be more productive. Then you could cross-check and sift the material and discuss and reflect on it over the next few years in groups, dyads, and by yourself.

You certainly don't have that kind of time—so we've done it for you.

In this book you'll be sitting down to a smorgasbord of ideas, insights, suggestions, solutions, workarounds, encouragement, and inspiration. But it's definitely a smorgasbord; we wouldn't expect anyone to eat all the dishes on the table, or even to sample all of them.

If you've been in practice 20 or 30 years, much of what you read here will probably get you nodding in agreement, "Yes, I've always thought that, but I've never seen it in print." You may find the old ideas familiar, but there are plenty of fresh suggestions that may be of great value to you (try the section on the winning style with patients in Part 4, or the "killer app" for clinical computing in Part 3).

If you're a new practitioner, you're probably already familiar with computers and patient satisfaction techniques. But the sections on clinical wisdom (Part 3) and colleague relationships (Part 4) may contain ideas that are new to you.

Whatever stage you're at in your career, you'll already be using some of the ideas in this book; some you've perhaps tried, but found unsuitable for your practice style, personality, or philosophy; some others won't make any sense to you at all.

But many of the ideas and suggestions will strike you as possible solutions to the real problems that you face every day in your practice. These can be pure gold.

So **use the feedback principle** by investing the time it takes you to read this book back into changing your daily practice. For instance, if you get through this book in four hours, and if you use just one idea out of the 140, and that idea saves you just 1/100th of your daily working time and effort—that will be a savings of 24 hours per year, or a *net annual profit on time invested of 500%.* Do you know of any other investment that can net you 500% annually?

## Using This Book Most Efficiently

Okay, you're a busy practitioner who needs to get the biggest and fastest return possible on your time and effort. This book is designed specifically to accommodate your needs. You'll find a minimum of theory and discussion, and a maximum of practical suggestions you can use *today* to make your professional life more efficient and more pleasant.

To use this book more efficiently, start with the brief self-diagnostic quiz (Exercise 1–1). Take two or three minutes to fill it out, being as honest as you can, but moving quickly through the questions, not laboring over them. Do that now, please, before you read on.

**Exercise 1–1**  Physician Productivity Self-Diagnostic Quiz

Directions: Please circle Y(es) or N(o) for each question, being as honest as you can.

1. I basically feel I don't have enough time.                                Y   N

2. My family would like to see more of me.                                Y   N

3. My practice just isn't much fun any more.     Y   N

4. I feel too exhausted to think, a lot of the time.     Y   N

5. My professional goal is just to keep working.     Y   N

6. My schedule is pretty much made up by my staff.     Y   N

7. My calendar keeps getting fuller.     Y   N

8. Part of my day is spent on garbage.     Y   N

9. I have a lot of unfinished projects.     Y   N

10. I guess I go to some meetings mainly out of habit.     Y   N

11. Frankly, I have too much paperwork.     Y   N

12. I'm interrupted pretty frequently at work.     Y   N

13. I tend to put some things off, and then have to rush.     Y   N

14. It's hard to locate papers, etc. in my own office.     Y   N

15. I basically leave my CME to the experts.     Y   N

16. I rarely (or never) use a PC in my clinical work.     Y   N

17. I can't keep up with the new knowledge in my field.     Y   N

18. To keep up, I mainly browse the journals.     Y   N

19. In my office is a pile of unread journals.   Y   N

20. Frankly, I'm too old to learn much new stuff.   Y   N

21. I'm too rushed to listen to patients' stories.   Y   N

22. Treatment decisions are basically my responsibility.   Y   N

23. I feel isolated from many of my colleagues.   Y   N

24. Others in my team cause a lot of friction.   Y   N

25. To get things done right, I have to be hard on people.   Y   N

## Scoring Your Self-Diagnostic Quiz

Add up your total Yes answers on the self-diagnostic quiz. At our seminars, most physicians have between 5 and 15 Yes answers. You've learned your first useful fact: You're not alone! We've all got problems these days.

If you've been candid and have 4 or fewer Yes answers, you're already very successful at self-management. We'd like to hear how you're doing it (you'll find mailing and e-mail addresses on the title page).

The main portion of this book is split into three sections (Parts 2, 3, and 4), roughly corresponding to groups of related questions on the self-diagnostic quiz. Each practitioner's pattern of Yes answers will be different, but if most of yours are clumped in the first 14 questions, you may be particularly interested in "Time Management for Physicians" (Part 2); if many of your Yes answers are between #15 and #20, you may want to focus on "Knowledge

Management for Physicians" (Part 3); if many of your Yes answers clumped between #21 and #25, you might give extra attention to "Relationship Management for Physicians" (Part 4).

As you read through this book, you'll find suggestions printed in **boldface type**. As you read, **mark the pages where you find useful suggestions or exercises** that make especially good sense for your practice at this time. Also, **download those suggestions you want to incorporate into your practice** by marking them on the lists at the end of each part headed "Suggestions I Will Try." You'll also find spaces there for you to jot down your own suggestions as they occur to you.

---

**Warning/Disclaimer:** *The author does not suggest you change your current clinical practice in any particular way; that would be presumptuous and possibly risky. Only you can safely judge which suggestions (if any) would be prudent and useful to try in your own professional work. This book is presented for information and entertainment only, not as a peer-reviewed textbook, and none of the material herein is meant to supplant any individual physician's judgment.*

---

Since I'm also still a student, I'd very much like to hear back from you about what works—and what doesn't—for you, and why. Also, you'll have your own ways of doing some things that are better than the suggestions in this book (in fact, every physician has his or her own individual way of being productive, efficient, and happy at work). Send us your observations and suggestions; I promise to pass on your practical techniques in a future edition.

Now let's get started by finding out what this productivity thing is all about.

## Notes

1. W. Osler, *Aequanimitas* (Philadelphia, PA: Blakiston, 1932), 423.
2. "MSOs, PPMs Help Physicians Navigate Managed Care," *Psychiatric Times*, August 1997, 33.
3. B. Jancin, "Rising Doctor Disability Claims Draw Scrutiny," *Clinical Psychiatry News*, December 1995, 5.
4. C. Quinn, "Computerized Records Put a Good Spin on Healthcare," *Managed Healthcare*, March 1997, 71–80.
5. "Managed Care Linked to Pay Dip for Docs," *Managed Healthcare*, October 1996, 16.

## ✦ 2 ✦

# What Is Physician Productivity?

So why is everyone suddenly so excited about productivity? We physicians haven't exactly been sitting on our hands all these years, have we?

No—in fact we've been very busy. Unfortunately, being busy doesn't necessarily translate into being productive. And productivity is a fateful issue for every American worker, including us. Without major increases in productivity, the likelihood that any industry or profession will successfully make it very far into the new century is, at best, questionable.

## We're Not As Efficient As We Think We Are

Management guru Peter Drucker wrote recently that the single greatest challenge facing managers in the developed countries of the world is to *raise the productivity of knowledge workers*.[1]

Who are these knowledge workers who need their productivity raised?

*We* are knowledge workers.

Huge investments have been made in our education, training, instruments, and in the trillion-dollar capital plant of buildings, machines, systems, and employees that we take for granted as our birthright.

However, it turns out that although knowledge workers may be highly intelligent, superbly trained, and well motivated, *we're simply not very efficient*. And this is as true of health care workers (including physicians) as it is of university professors, engineers, and attorneys. Studies have concluded that the U.S. health care system generally runs at between 40% and 60% efficiency.[2] In other words, about half of what we do is wasted, and produces no effective return on investment of resources and effort. (If this sounds low, consider that the internal combustion engine, after 100 years of engineering, is only about 10% efficient.) So Drucker is at least half right: There's plenty of room for improvement.

New clinical knowledge, new treatment methods, new technology, new organizational arrangements, and new financial structures are making our profession over. All of these changes dictate that we rethink the traditional ways of practicing and look for ways to become more efficient at everything we do.

As I write this, 9 of 10 physicians being recruited are eligible for some sort of productivity bonus,[3] while patient satisfaction and retention have become fiscal incentives for the 90% of U.S. physicians who deal with managed care.[4,5]

At the same time, physician reimbursement is going down, so most practitioners are finding they have to speed up just to stay even; the average primary care visit is down from 15 minutes in the 1980s to only 10 minutes—and headed lower.[6] At the same time, physicians whose patients complain about them can find themselves deselected (i.e., fired).

In short, we're getting whipsawed between (1) the need to work faster and cheaper, and (2) the need to do higher quality work that meets our patients' expectations. Since no physician wants to reduce quality of care, we're forced to find ways to be more productive and efficient while still being effective.

## Who Can Manage Physicians?

The question really isn't whether we're going to become more efficient and productive, but rather how we're going to accomplish this.

### MANAGERS

Drucker implies that external managers can somehow make individual knowledge workers more efficient. While this sounds logical, no one has ever been able to prove it. It turns out that trying to manage autonomous–creative–scientific professionals such as engineers, chemists, and doctors is a lot like herding cats. Want to see how useless it is to manage an independent craftsman doing a procedure you don't fully understand? Try it the next time a plumber is working on your pipes.

Medical directors and other physician-managers usually (and quite rightly) don't get too involved with an individual doctor's unique practice patterns; they tend to focus more on global and systemic changes.

### CONSULTANTS

Cartoon someone stuck on my door: A prosperous-looking consultant is pulling a huge book out of his briefcase and handing it across the desk to a frazzled doc. The consultant is saying, "And this 500-page procedures manual will simplify your practice." Right.

Consultants' and practice management experts' newest solutions for inefficiencies in health care include practice guidelines, disease management systems, critical pathways, care maps, computerized scheduling, CQI, TQM, and dozens of similar systems-based approaches. Anything that will make our offices and hospitals run more smoothly is welcome, and the sudden efflorescence of so many new wrinkles is a good sign: It shows we're a profession and an industry in full transition into the new millennium. However, it's hard to tell how many of these innovations will survive; they tend to be rushed to market with a lot of fanfare and not much research. Some on the list may already be out of favor by the time you read this.

## Managed Care and Our More Efficient Future

However, one group of methods for making health care more efficient has demonstrated astonishing success: managed care.

Managed care actually means managing costs—for the employer or insurance company who is paying the bills. Mostly by controlling patients' access to services, encouraging competition among providers for access to patients, discounting and capitating, and the like, managed care organizations (MCOs) routinely are able to take 20%–30% off the top for their administrative costs and profit. This leaves providers to figure out how to provide optimum patient care with whatever is left over. It's crude, but it works.

MCOs simply assume that if anyone can make health care more efficient, we, the practitioners, can. In this they're correct: 90% of health care costs are generated in the direct administration and delivery of care.[7] As a result of its success up to now at lowering the costs of health care, managed care has become popular with corporations, consumers, and politicians in a very short time.

As I write this, however, some of the country's health care giants are hemorrhaging red ink, undergoing investigation for possible criminal activities, holding off striking nurses, or worse. Many states are preparing legislation that will regulate MCOs, expose them to malpractice risk, liberalize access to providers, and scrutinize quality of care. Meanwhile, physicians and hospitals are starting to form provider groups large enough to negotiate service contracts directly with employers (whether this approach will be as successful as fourth-party managed care isn't yet clear).

It's always impossible to see the future; most people who claim to be making predictions are just indulging in wishful thinking or propaganda. But it does seem that for the foreseeable future, corporations—who are dictating cuts in health care costs—will continue to have their way because they pay the bills. Employee groups (patients) who might be demanding freer access and more benefits have lost some of their clout. Competition and cost-cutting in health care are not going away.

The bottom line: Whether mandated by MCOs, by government payers, or by our own practice groups, increased speed and efficiency of health care delivery are here to stay. And while some speedup and savings can be produced by systems fixes, in the end it's up to the individual practitioner to make his or her practice more efficient.

> ❝Managing care from the outside-in... involves...restructuring, offering financial rewards and penalties, and so on....But for someone working in the front line of medical care, dealing with patients day-to-day, the inside-out approach is much more powerful.❞
>
> John Wisniewsky, MD, MHSA
> Director, Henry Ford Health System
> Managed Care College[8(p.5)]

Let's be clear: We're not going back—not to house calls by horse and buggy, and not to the cottage-industry, unregulated fee-for-service medicine of our youth. While the past is over, the future of medicine is still very bright—but it's a future in which every physician will have to compete by being maximally efficient and effective.

Therefore, one of the goals of this book is to equip the best-trained, most able, and most ethical practitioners to compete more effectively—and stay in the game.

## Self-Management Makes Sense

A promising approach to increasing professionals' efficiency and productivity is laid out in the management literature: Simply put, you must **start managing yourself** to be more efficient and effective at what you do. Self-management for physicians means that you take charge of crucial areas of your professional life; you no longer allow others to dictate how you prioritize your time, acquire your clinical knowledge, and structure your professional relationships. You work lean and strip the waste out of your clinical functions. Streamlined, efficient practices are in less danger from competition, takeovers, stagnation, and other perils.

Other industries are also turning to self-management by professionals to increase efficiency. One airline now lets its professional flight crews use a bank of computers to check in and out, file their logs, and communicate. No managers are involved. It seems to work fine, and it saves money.

In the main, we physicians would also prefer to manage ourselves. External management means less autonomy and more expense—somebody has to pay salaries and bonuses for all those health care managers, consultants, marketers, information specialists, vice presidents, and CEOs—and they don't work cheap. Also, self-management and continuous self-improvement come naturally to us docs.

Unfortunately, up to now there have been no good texts or courses on even the rudiments of physician self-management. In fact, although there are 240 books in print on time management, e.g., for everyone from hairdressers to CEOs, there's not a single one written specifically for physicians.

This book tries to fill that gap and meet the need for a practical guide for physicians who want to hone their skills of personal self-management. Authored by a full-time practitioner with 30 years of experience, and based on suggestions made by other busy clinicians, this book is written from the inside of the profession (so it's on your side), and starts with the premise that we physicians are willing and able to manage ourselves.

All the suggestions contained in these pages have been used by successful practitioners, and can be put into practice immediately by any physician, without making costly changes in systems, hardware, staff structures, and the like.

## Physician Productivity: What It Isn't

A physician jumped up at this point in a seminar and demanded, "Who says we're only 60% efficient? Do they understand what we actually do, much less whether or not we're productive?"

It's true that a lot of nonsense is being written these days about productivity; the word itself can have many meanings, depending on the writer's point of view. Economists use a standard definition of productivity for industrial workers, represented by the first equation in Figure 2–1.

You can see from the first equation that the productivity (P) of a worker producing widgets is equal to the total number of widgets she makes (her output), divided by the input (which is usually time spent on the job)—or, more simply, *widgets per hour.*

This first equation has the advantage of simplicity, but it takes for granted several conditions:

✦ The only thing this worker does every day is make widgets.
✦ Every widget is pretty much like every other widget.
✦ Society needs a lot of identical widgets made quickly.

Industrial worker (widget maker, e.g.):

$$P = \frac{Outputs}{Inputs} = \frac{Widgets}{Time\ worked} = Widgets\ per\ hour$$

Knowledge worker (physician, e.g.):

$$P = \frac{(Appropriate\ outcomes) - (Inappropriate\ outcomes)}{(Effective\ inputs) + (Ineffective\ inputs)} \times C \times R$$

**Figure 2–1** Productivity (P) for two types of workers.

✦ Broken or damaged widgets don't really matter (just throw 'em in the broken-widget pail).
✦ The widget maker will do nothing but make identical widgets for her entire working life.

This first equation could apply as well to robots as to human workers—and in fact has been so applied.

Well, my friend, one thing should be obvious to you...*We don't make widgets!*

## Physician Productivity Is Different

Productivity in the healing professions is significantly different from robots making widgets, even if some health care analysts seem to ignore this fact.

For obvious starters, like all service workers, *we work with, for, and through people,* not on machines that crank out widgets. Without sick and injured people, there's no reason to have doctors.

Also, *what we actually do is much more complex* than making widgets or servicing gadgets. Even flying an airworthy 747 is less complex than what we do: Most of our days are spent fixing sick or injured patients, complex biologic systems that by definition *are always crashing*.

Another crucial difference between us and the widget makers is that we physicians actually own and control our own tools. This fact will be explained in detail later, but suffice to say now that this allows us to increase our personal productivity radically.

Now let's study for a moment the second equation in Figure 2–1, which may give a clearer idea of what physician productivity really is.

## Is This Outcome Appropriate?

Above the line, in the numerator, is the basic service rendered by physicians: "appropriate outcomes." This seems quite obvious at first; when we do an indicated procedure, prescribe an effective medication, or interact therapeutically with an ill or injured patient, we're achieving an appropriate outcome—aren't we?

Maybe. In the past few years everything has gotten more complicated, including this once-simple concept. For instance, if you've performed the indicated procedure flawlessly and achieved an excellent technical outcome (from your point of view) but the patient is wildly unhappy with the care he has received and wants to sue you—is that an appropriate or an inappropriate outcome?

Since we're in the service sector, all of our outcomes are co-produced with other people (most usually, our patients); that's what the "R" in the equation reminds us. We never really work alone, and we never produce an output without at least one other human being in the relationship.

In this era of "entitled demanders," knee-jerk malpractice suits, and MCO customer satisfaction surveys, outcomes are becoming a very hot issue, and we'll try to get some guidance in Part 4. For now, suffice to say that appropriate outcomes are the main product we're seeking to maximize, so it belongs in the numerator of our productivity equation.

Mark that our main product is always optimal clinical outcomes—not dollars, not cost savings, not profits. We need to be on guard these days; people will try to confuse us about this crucial issue if they can get away with it. For instance, a celebrated health care economist recently wrote, "[P]atients can be viewed as biological structures that will yield future cash flows."[9(p.1,850)] This statement was published in our leading medical journal— and without any editorial comment. But as clinicians and as professionals, we can't possibly agree with this point of view.

For us, why does the provision of optimal medical care outweigh the profit motive every time?

Most simply and obviously, *because in the clinical encounter, when our patient is sick or bleeding or dying, lifesaving medical care is what's important to them—not profits!*

And we work for our patient, always. If we don't, who will?

### "The Golden Scalpel"

It was a melodramatic 1950s thriller in the medicine-money-sex genre, but somehow I still remember the plot of a book that went from hand to hand when I was in medical school.

The yarn went something like this (my apologies to the author): Two surgeons were practicing at the same hospital, one of them capable but somewhat weak-willed, and the other a sleazy bungler who routinely butchered every patient he cut on. Because big profits were involved, the first doctor covered up for his incompetent partner, who continued to mess up his surgical patients.

Because he was making so much money from the arrangement, the first doctor was not moved by the pain and suffering of his partner's patients, nor by the pleas of his colleagues, and would do nothing about his partner's incompetence. Then one day he himself was injured seriously in an auto accident, and required major surgery.

As the book ends, the first doctor is lying injured, helpless, and unable to speak on a gurney, about to be rolled into the OR. He looks up and sees, to his horror, leaning over him and about to perform surgery on him...his incompetent butcher of a partner.

A bit pulpy, perhaps, but it reminded us of a very basic truth: No one goes through life without eventually needing urgent health care for themselves or their family. We have to make sure it won't be second best.

Every physician is intimately acquainted with the negative term in the numerator, "inappropriate outcomes." No matter what we do—and, rarely, *because* of what we do or fail to do—a certain percentage of our patients will not improve, will get worse, or will die. Every physician desperately wants to keep these inappropriate outcomes to a minimum.

These are not just broken widgets; these are broken tissues, broken organs, broken lives.

Large parts of this book are devoted to helping you decrease poor outcomes: Time management gives you more time to do proper care; knowledge management lets you apply the latest and most effective skills and knowledge when and where they can do the most good; and relationship management can make all your patient and staff contacts more likely to promote healing, while ensuring that the people doing your work for you are also maximally effective.

## Cutting Down Our Inputs

Looking at the denominator, we can see that both input terms need to be reduced as far as possible, since they're added together and divided into the numerator. The term on the left of the denominator, "effective inputs," is the sum of all the time, mental and physical effort, judgment, technical skill, knowledge, observation, human contact, training, communicating, etc., that we put in to produce outcomes. In other words, it's what the resource-based relative value system (RBRVS) was supposed to be based on.[10]

Because they're in the denominator, effective inputs need to be reduced as much as is feasible—but plainly there are minimum levels below which we start giving worse care, and the effort becomes self-defeating. For example, if we try to see too many patients and cut down our input of time per patient, our rate of both errors and patient dissatisfaction (inappropriate outcomes) may go up, and our diagnostic precision (appropriate outcomes) may drop. If we try to rush our way through a laparoscopic common bile duct exploration, we may get a perforation (inappropriate outcome).

What we can do is make these appropriate inputs as efficient as possible. In Part 2 we'll show how getting control of your schedule can free up time for more procedures and patient visits. In Part 3 we'll become more efficient at managing our personal clinical knowledge base, so that we're better and quicker at acquiring and updating the skills we need to do the job. In Part 4 we'll describe some techniques for speeding up the rate at which we see patients, while still giving concentrated attention to each one.

Our own inputs are only part of this equation. As we'll see also in Part 4, if we have efficient and dedicated staff, cooperative patients, and helpful colleagues, then all our work becomes much more effective and satisfying.

Research indicates, however, that the biggest hindrance to the efficiency of knowledge workers is actually the second term in the denominator, "ineffective inputs." In plain English, that's wasted time and effort. For example:

✦ You can't locate your patient's history (or lab work or x-ray report) just at the moment you need it to make a crucial decision.
✦ You have to stop work early and spend 30 minutes catching up on paperwork.
✦ You wait around 45 minutes for an operating room.
✦ You find yourself sitting in a useless meeting.
✦ You attend a workshop and realize you're already familiar with the subject matter.
✦ You spend 10 minutes on the phone with a patient, and finally just tell her to come to the office to see you.
✦ You have to spend an hour meeting with your staff to iron out a series of misunderstandings, patient incidents, poor communications, and the like.

But you can make your own list of how your time and effort get wasted every single day.

You'll find dozens of ideas throughout this book for reducing your wasted inputs (and inappropriate outcomes) to a minimum; decreasing these terms are the secret of increasing your productivity dramatically.

If you look around you, you'll see that many physicians are terribly busy doing a lot of the stuff on the bottom line of the equation, maximizing their inputs. They're always rushing, always pushing, often stressed. But what finally counts is not how much you input, it's what comes out on the top line of the equation—that is, the quality and quantity of your outcomes.

In other words, the bottom line of the equation is how busy you are, but the top line indicates how *productive* you are.

Take a moment to study the physician productivity equation. If you understand it, you can pretty much figure out what you need to do to increase your personal productivity, at least in the short term.

## Medical Careers and Working Relationships

But if you've been in medicine for any significant length of time, you know there are at least two more terms that need to be figured into the equation.

"C" is the Career factor—physicians, unlike widget makers, aren't in it for the short run. Medicine is uniquely a lifetime calling. *Ars longa, vita breva.* We doctors often have spent almost half our lives learning medicine before we ever see our first paying patient.

So we need to think about our lifelong productivity: How can we sustain our motivation and enthusiasm over 30 or 40 years of practice? How will we deal with the inevitable changes in medicine as we grow older in the profession? What will happen to our productivity as we become older? The answers to these questions figure in our total productivity.

In any service profession, no one works alone. "R" in the equation symbolizes our relationships with our patients, our teams, and our colleagues. Our productivity depends to a great extent on how well we form and maintain these relationships. We'll devote all of Part 4 to optimizing this crucial term in the productivity equation.

## Every Physician Uses the Same Basic Tools

A few months ago, I was looking out the back window of our house when I saw some workmen arrive on the property next door to start excavating what would eventually be a horse corral. Equipped only with shovels, they scraped away for several hours, without making much of a dent. Then, around noon, a fellow drove up with a trailer carrying a huge bulldozer. He went to work,

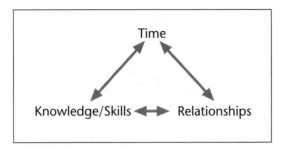

**Figure 2–2** The physician's three basic tools.

---

and in a few hours he moved more dirt with his 'dozer than the crew with the shovels could have moved in several weeks.

What made that man so productive?

Sure—he had the right tool for the job, and he knew how to use it.

We physicians don't bring a bulldozer to work with us in the morning (some mornings we probably wish we did). But we do bring some basic tools. Our tools turn out to be three in number (Figure 2–2):

1. *Time:* If we don't put in time at our profession, our productivity is automatically zero.
2. *Knowledge and skills:* Webster's definition of practice is "application of knowledge." By applying knowledge over time in our practice, we produce all our outcomes.
3. *Relationships:* We all work for, with, and through people.

Whether we also use a laparoscope or a tongue blade, whether we work on salary for Permanente in a huge metropolis or run a solo office in rural eastern Oregon, whether we practice in front of a teleradiology monitor from our castle in Ireland or out of a rucksack in a mud hut in Zimbabwe—these are our three basic tools, and we all use them, every working moment of our professional lives.

## How the Three Tools Synergize

These three tools reinforce each other. For instance, consider the brand-new first-year resident on her first day of work.

She comes on the floor at seven in the morning, and is immediately thrown into a wild scene of rounds, admissions, procedures, decisions, emergencies, outpatient appointments, and so on. She has plenty of general clinical knowledge from medical school, but little of the practical, specialized knowledge she'll need to be adept at her new specialty. And she has no clue about using her tools in an optimal way: How long should a procedure take? Who will help her? Who should she avoid? Who can she call for fast advice when she needs it? What needs to be done first? Next? What scut can she delegate? Where's the equipment she needs? Where's the chart? *Where's the restroom?*

No wonder residents often report that when they finish their first day on the job, usually in the early hours of the next morning, they just go somewhere and throw up from the stress.

Same resident, a year or two later: She comes on the floor with full confidence, because she knows exactly what she'll be doing and how long it will take her, what needs to be checked immediately and what she can let go till she has a moment, and what unexpected things can be expected (Time); what specialized knowledge she really needs for this job and how to get it fastest, and from whom, in her personal network (Knowledge); whom she'll work with, how to get others to do her work for her, and whom she can't trust to do anything right (Relationships). She's gotten so efficient that she probably is able to knock off early and catch an hour of TV in the residents' lounge.

So what do we call her now?

Fully trained.

Actually, she hasn't really gained much didactic knowledge (although she's picked up a lot of practical, specialized knowledge in her field), and she's putting in much less time—but she has learned how to use these tools efficiently, and leverage both of them through her working relationships.

Another example: If you're working with MCOs, you know that ramping up the tempo of your clinical schedule so you can see more patients in less time is necessary (I didn't say it was good, or right—just necessary). But you also know that to make your limited time spent on each clinical contact more productive, cutting out inefficient work habits is a must, as is having a more quickly available knowledge and information base, as well as smoother working relationships with colleagues and co-workers.

As you read this book and try the exercises in self-analysis, you'll become conscious of how well you use the three tools of our profession, and from here on—for the rest of your professional life—you'll be aware of using these tools throughout every working day, so that you can keep analyzing your work habits and improving your efficiency indefinitely.

Economists teach that investment in our tools increases productivity (someone had to invest a chunk of money in my neighbor's bulldozer). By investing a small amount of time and effort in thinking about your work habits, you can become much more productive—and maintain and increase that productivity for the rest of your working life.

The mark of an excellent craftsperson is the consummate skill with which she uses the tools of her craft. But these skills of time, knowledge, and relationship management are not taught in medical school or residency. As far as I know, this is the only book that discusses these three subjects expressly for physicians.

> ❝You don't get better at doing something unless you stop to think about what you've been doing— to analyze the process.❞
>
> Michael Doyle and David Straus[11(p.19)]

Enough theory.

Our approach is basically a practical one, stressing acquisition of new attitudes and methods.

"Attitudes? Why attitudes?" you ask. Because they decide how we see our world, how we feel, and how we do our work. Most of our attitudes are unconscious, so we never question them, much less change them. In talking with hundreds of physicians since 1993, one thing that has struck me is how many outdated attitudes we all carry around from medical school and training—probably because that was when we were most impressionable and learned the most about being doctors.

Just a few examples of attitude baggage that we picked up in med school and training, and which we never question:

- ✦ It's more efficient if other people arrange my schedule for me.
- ✦ Teachers know best what I need to learn, and how to teach it to me.
- ✦ Being smart and technically proficient is more important than cultivating good professional relationships.
- ✦ To be fast and efficient, I can't get hung up spending time with patients and co-workers (almost all residents learn this one).

We'll soon see how these and other outdated attitudes sap our productivity, and we'll make some concrete suggestions for acquiring new, more appropriate ways of looking at our professional work.

The first new attitude we want you to acquire is that **you definitely can improve your efficiency**. Other physicians like you have done it already. I have done it. You'll find in this book more than 140 concrete suggestions for doing it. So you definitely can do it.

In fact, just adopting this can-do attitude will guarantee that you'll look for—and find—ways to be more efficient.

So now let's start learning in detail some techniques for using more effectively the tools of our craft in order to become more productive physicians. We'll start with the biggest bugaboo for every practitioner: Time.

---

**Notes**

1. P.F. Drucker, "The New Productivity Challenge," *The Harvard Business Review*, November–December 1991, 69–79.
2. A.B. Godfrey, Interview, *Quality Connection*, Summer 1994, 2.
3. "Study Shows That 60% of Physicians Are Recruited as Salaried Employees," *Managed Healthcare*, August 1996, 58.
4. "Percent of Physicians with Managed Care Contracts in 1996," *Clinical Psychiatry News*, July 1997, 1.
5. "A Portrait of Managed Care Practice," *Clinical Psychiatry News*, April 1995, 10.
6. C. Quinn, "Computerized Records Put a Good Spin on Healthcare," *Managed Healthcare*, March 1997, 71–80.
7. Quinn, p. 72.
8. J. Wisniewsky, "Continuous Improvement in Physician Education," *IHI Quality Connection*, Spring 1997, 5.
9. U.E. Reinhardt, "Economics," *Journal of the American Medical Association* 277, no. 23 (1997): 1,850–1,851.
10. W.C. Hsiao et al., "Resource Based Relative Values," *Journal of the American Medical Association* 260, no. 16 (1988): 2,347–2,353.
11. M. Doyle and D. Straus, *How to Make Meetings Work* (New York: Playboy, 1977), 19.

# Part 2

# Time Management
# for Physicians

"We are our calendar."

Tom Peters[1](p.498)

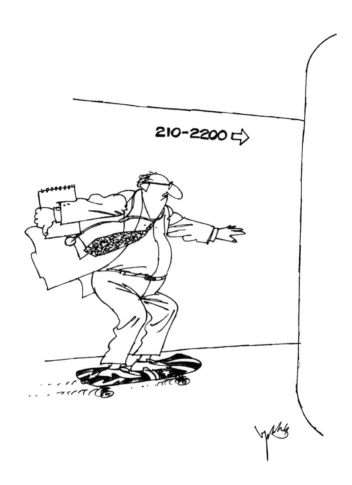

# ✦ 3 ✦

# Two Crucial
# First Steps

When speaking before an audience of physicians and their spouses, I always ask, "Please raise your hand if you wish your doctor-husband or -wife could spend more time with you." Almost every other hand in the room goes up. (For fun, I also ask, "Now raise your hand if you'd rather see *less* of your doctor-husband or -wife." Occasionally, a few hands do go up!)

Survey after survey shows that "not enough time" is most doctors' biggest complaint. As one harried ophthalmologist put it, "I don't even have time to think any more!" If you personally do not feel your hours are too long, try asking your family how they feel about it.

The average physician is putting in about 58 hours per week at his or her profession (including travel, paperwork, meetings, continuing education, and other chores).[2] As managed care becomes pervasive, busy practitioners are reporting that 80-hour weeks are not unusual ("I'm my own boss—I can work any 80 hours of the week I choose"). Many of us work the "eight-day week," testing the limits of what any professional can be expected to handle.

At a seminar in San Francisco I asked a large group of surgeons, "What will you do as reimbursements keep going down and competition keeps going up?" Their surprising reply: "We'll just work harder."

I don't think that's the right answer.

## Working Longer and Harder Is Not the Solution

We're already pushing the envelope of how much time and effort we can put in and still be productive, accurate, and sane practitioners—not to speak of the effect on our families. Also, working longer hours leaves us less time for planning, training, and reflecting—and so decreases our long-term efficiency.

No, we really don't want to work longer or harder. But doing less than is necessary for our patients, giving them lower quality care, just isn't an option for us either. So we want to work smarter —which basically means getting rid of less useful tasks and getting more from each hour of work.

Here are dozens of practical suggestions from busy, successful physicians for working the same or fewer hours, but getting better results, and more personal satisfaction, from every minute of our working day:

## The Surprising First Step

First, **choose a personal professional goal**.

This probably seems counterintuitive, or irrelevant; you're asking, "What does choosing a professional goal have to do with managing my time?" A whole lot, as it turns out.

I've found that very few physicians actually have any goal. In a typical seminar audience of a hundred or so doctors, usually only three or four hands go up when I ask how many have a written, discrete goal that they're working on in their professional life.

Yet being "self-actualizing"—choosing your own goals, working on them, and achieving them—is one of three factors that have predicted outstanding professional success in physicians. (The other two predictors were high intellectual interest and executive ability—we'll get to those in Parts 3 and 4.)

In contrast to doctors, all managers have goals. The shop foreman has a goal of turning out so many widgets per week, the plant manager has a quarterly quota to make, the company CEO is working on a 5- or even a 20-year plan. In Japan, corporate CEOs often have 100-year goals. If you're a manager, the higher up the corporate ladder you go, the more crucial it is to have goals, and the longer time horizon your goals cover.

Managers criticize physicians on this one, calling us "15-minute docs." They describe our work patterns as "discontinuous"—in other words, endlessly repeating days and years cut up into 10-minute or 15-minute patient visits, with no broad, long-term purpose in view.

Why don't physicians have personal professional goals?

I think it starts with our education and training. For the first 30 years of our lives, we don't have to set any goals; someone else is always doing it for us. The first goal was the high school GPA we needed to get into a good college, then the college grades we needed for med school, then the recommendations we needed to get a first-rate residency, then enough training and experience and cramming to pass our boards. All these goals were laid out so neatly and clearly that most of us probably never even thought about choosing a personal goal, shooting for something we wanted to do on our own.

That was then. Now, no one else is going to set your goals for you—nor should they. Only you can say what direction you want to go in your professional life.

If you take a few minutes here and now to set yourself a personal professional goal, it can change your life more than any other single idea in this book. Let me try to convince you.

## No Goal Means No Rudder

Near our home in northern California is San Francisco Bay, a mecca for sailing yachts. On a clear, breezy day, you can see these white-hulled beauties racing out on the water. At the blast of a cannon they plunge off down the wind, spinnakers billowing, spray flying, heeling over as they tack tightly around the buoys and churn through the whitecaps for the finish line. A yacht race is a sight for the gods to see!

Now imagine those same yachts racing on the bay—but without a rudder. The cannon would go off—*crack!*—and they'd tear out into the bay, and there'd be a lot of dashing around, back and forth, spray flying, and they'd cover a lot of water, but at the end of the race they wouldn't have sailed anywhere, just in aimless circles...or even under the Golden Gate Bridge and out into the trackless Pacific.

If we don't have a goal, we don't have a rudder.

We may be doing a lot of rushing, churning up a lot of spray, going at top speed, dashing back and forth—but in the end, we haven't really gotten anywhere.

And at the end of the day—at the end of all our days—we may ask ourselves, plaintively, "Is this really what I wanted to do with my professional life? Is this what I went to school 24 years for? Were there other things in medicine I wanted to accomplish?"

Lack of professional goals may explain that familiar phenomenon, the excellent physician who, at 45 or 50 years old, suddenly develops a consuming interest in mutual funds, or winemaking, or multilevel marketing. Practicing medicine no longer holds much of a challenge or sense of accomplishment for him. In this way we lose some of our best and most seasoned practitioners.

## Something to Look Forward To

Human nature is such that everyone needs something to look forward to, or life gets painfully humdrum. We look forward to something all the time, even if it's just the weekend—how would you feel if someone told you there wouldn't be any more weekends; that from now on, you'd just work without ever stopping?

Doctors, because we spend so much of our youth putting off personal gratification, are especially future oriented, and definitely need to look forward to some reward or achievement.

This explains how we were able to work such long hours during our training. Remember for a moment those shining autumn days when you were starting med school, and it was all in front of you. Chances are, the thrill of expectation made the grueling seven-day weeks of studying not only bearable, but fun. And as residents, we always had June 30th to look forward to.

One reason our long schedules make us depressed and exhausted is that now we see no end in sight. Many practitioners feel they're on an endless treadmill of 14-hour days and frequent nights on call, with no goal except eventually to retire when they're worn out (if they're lucky), or die in harness (if they're not).

To raise our morale while we work, we need to have some kind of goal in our professional lives, something we can look forward to...with pleasure.

## A Goal Sets Our Priorities

We have competing demands from all sides: our patients, our office and hospital staffs, our colleagues, and our families are all pushing for a place on our calendar. We know we can't possibly do it all. Take out that set of index cards or (electronic) datebook you carry in your breast pocket with all your work listed on it and look at it. Did it ever occur to you that you'll probably still have a bunch of stuff on your cards that you haven't done when they carry you off to the mortuary?

Since we can't possibly do everything, having a goal lets us know every minute what's important to us, and what we can dump.

For example, here's something that happens a lot, if you're a busy practitioner: You find yourself with 30 minutes of available time before starting a procedure. But you have important phone calls, some pressing paperwork, an overdue discussion with a co-worker, and one or two other urgent matters. If you have only enough time to do one thing, trying to decide which to do (or trying to do them all fast) will just stress you. But if you have a personal goal—one that you've chosen in a cool moment of self-analysis—you automatically **prioritize the one activity that most closely relates to your goal**. Simple. No time wasted in trying to decide what to do next. No guilt. No stress. No pressure.

> **"**[A] long life without the feeling of fulfillment is very tedious.**"**
>
> Hans Selye, MD[3(p.438)]

When I decided to take my specialty boards at age 50, I knew I'd have to get in a certain amount of studying in order to pass. Having that goal changed my priorities. For about six months before the written exam, I filled every spare moment during my workday with studying and reviewing. At night, I didn't watch any TV unless I had completed two hours of study (I didn't miss anything). By the end of the six months, I was studying when I went to the bathroom. Having an important goal prioritized my time; it also challenged me to stretch myself, and it made me much more interested in my clinical work.

### A Goal Makes Progress Measurable

If you have a real goal, you can check every day to see if you're getting closer to your final objective; this gives you a tangible feeling that you're getting somewhere, no matter how small each daily increment may be. If you have no goal, days and months and even years can slip away, with no sense of having accomplished anything definite.

> **❝Time spent not getting where you want to go, no matter how efficiently you might not be getting there, is time wasted.❞**
>
> Stephanie Winston[4(p.205)]

Importantly, when you work toward your own goal, you get back control of part of your professional life. The deep satisfaction that comes from having accomplished something daily, of moving steadily forward, will definitely decrease your stress level. When your work is goal-directed, you'll be more likely to find yourself "in the flow." If you do some work on your personal goal first thing each day, no matter what unexpected delays and frustrations hit you later—even the dreaded 6 PM emergency admission—you can stay relaxed, knowing you've already accomplished your personal work.

In sum, having a personal professional goal will give you:

✦ some definite direction in your daily working life and your career

✦ a sense of personal control and autonomy, which will make you more focused and more relaxed

✦ something pleasant to look forward to, thereby raising your morale and adding some spice to your professional life

✦ a sure-fire way to prioritize your busy schedule, eliminating the stress of deciding what to do next, or trying to do it all

✦ after a few years, a sense of achievement that will increase your personal satisfaction by 100% (at least).

## Do It Now

So please leave off reading for a few minutes and think deeply about a personal professional goal that you would like to accomplish. Not just meeting the mortgage payments or paying your kids' college tuition (those are family duties, not personal goals) —make it something you want to do for your own professional growth, something that will mark a milestone in your further progress as a physician.

It should be important to you, achievable (a Nobel is probably out for most of us practitioners), yet something that calls on your powers—a "stretch goal." It should be something concrete that you can measure your progress toward in definite, yes/no steps (objectives), and also something you can achieve in a reasonable length of time (one to three years is the usual, or else it gets too abstract—but remember the Japanese).

These days, more physicians choose "adaptive" goals—projects that can help them weather our profession's massive changes: computers, new procedures/treatments, networking, and the like.

Some goals that busy physicians have chosen:

- ✦ taking the next step in their training (subspecialty boards, a ticket to do a special procedure, a mini-residency)
- ✦ moving to a new location
- ✦ reengineering their practice
- ✦ becoming adept at using personal computers in their clinical work
- ✦ becoming a consultant or locally acknowledged expert in their field
- ✦ learning another language to use in their practice
- ✦ paying back their loans (and/or their parents)
- ✦ taking a sabbatical year off
- ✦ publishing a piece of clinical research or case report

✦ earning an academic title
✦ getting an MBA or other administrative training
✦ increasing their annual practice income to a certain level

But beware of this last one: If you work persistently on a goal, you'll usually get it. So you'll want to pick your goal more carefully than the young practitioner I know who succeeded in getting her volume and income up after a few years. She now finds she's working very long hours seeing too many patients, because she didn't do what she really wanted—which was to develop and build a smaller practice around an exotic procedure at which she excels.

Or if you have "retirement" as your goal—as written, that's just a pipe dream. But "retire in X years with Y dollars" is a discrete, measurable goal, and you can see your progress toward it every day.

What if you can't think of a personal goal? Perhaps your practice is rolling along, and you're pretty satisfied with how things are going. One young generalist came forward after a seminar with just this question. After we talked for a few minutes, it became clear that he was a creative physician, with some dynamite ideas about how to do things in a completely new way. I encouraged him to take as his goal putting these radical innovations into practice, and I sincerely hope he will—he could single-handedly change the way we all work in the new century.

So if you're pretty satisfied with how things are going for yourself, maybe you can do something for others.

Now that you've taken a few minutes to think about and choose your goal, write it down. Why? Because it needs to be in a form you can read to yourself every day and that is clear, fixed, permanent, and not wishy-washy (the mind can play amazing tricks). If you have an index card handy, use that; if not, use Figure 3–1 and copy it later onto a card you can carry. Write your goal above the horizontal line on the index card, and then fill in the objectives or first steps toward your goal on

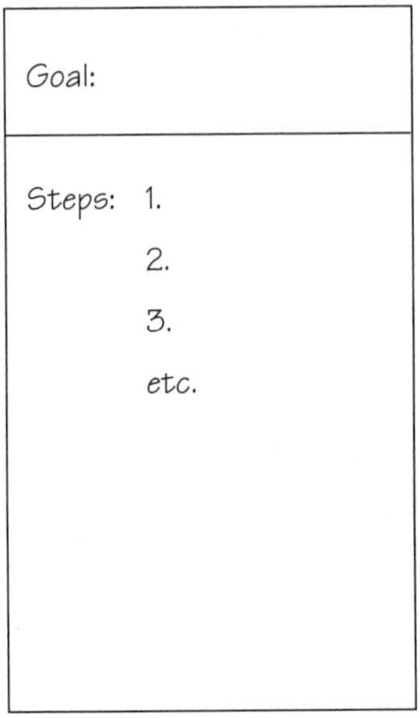

```
┌─────────────────────────────┐
│                             │
│  Goal:                      │
│                             │
├─────────────────────────────┤
│                             │
│  Steps:   1.                │
│                             │
│           2.                │
│                             │
│           3.                │
│                             │
│           etc.              │
│                             │
│                             │
│                             │
│                             │
│                             │
│                             │
└─────────────────────────────┘
```

**Figure 3–1** Your goal card.

the rest of that side of the card. (Leave the back of the card blank—we'll be using that side later.)

## Do Your Own Work First

If you pick up any book on getting rich through investing, it will say the secret is to *pay yourself first*. In other words, put aside a fixed amount of income every month toward your own investments—and do it before you pay anyone else. Paying everyone else first means you'll never have a penny left to invest, and you'll retire on a meager amount. If you're anywhere near retirement age, you know this maxim is true, and it's been worth a whole lot of money to you if you put it into effect early enough.

We need to apply exactly the same psychological tactic to achieving our personal professional goal: **work on your per-**

**sonal goal first thing every day**. Gradually, but definitely, you will achieve what you want. (Then you can choose a new goal.)

A young resident came to the lectern after a seminar at a university hospital. "I heard what you said about working on our own stuff every day, but with my schedule I just can't find the time to get my reading done. I know if I can't read while I'm still a resident, I'll probably never read."

I agreed with him on the importance of reading in his specialty, and asked him, "So what do you do first thing in the morning?"

"Well, I'm here at 6:30 to get ready for rounds—from then on it's solid."

"OK, what do you do between 5 and 6 in the morning?"

"Nothing. Sleep."

"That's when you should read. Between 5 and 6 AM. Every day."

The resident wrote me a few months later to say he had taken my advice, was reading something every morning (he went to bed a bit earlier), and was sailing happily through his residency.

Like you, I also have a demanding practice with very ill patients who require my full attention every working day, so a large part of this book is being written down at odd hours. As I write this chapter, in fact, I'm still in pajamas, finishing my morning cup of coffee. Completing this book is my goal for the year, so I'm careful to get some work done on it *every single day*. If you're holding this book in your hands, it's proof that this simple but powerful system worked again.

## Become a Card-Carrying Member

I said before that of all the ideas you'll find in this book, putting just this one into practice will change your professional life. In fact, no matter what else you try or don't try, if you've written down your professional goal on a card, if you carry it with you daily (one physician called it "joining the white card club"), and work on it religiously—I guarantee that in two or three years you will have accomplished something significant in your life that you might otherwise never have done.

You'll then have that steady, inner glow of personal satisfaction and confidence that comes when you accomplish something major, something above and beyond the normal grind. And according to researchers, increased self-esteem is one of the highest indicators of how happy people are.

So try it. Become a card-carrying member of the club right now. You can't possibly lose anything (except the price of an index card)—and you have a great deal to gain. In future years you may have forgotten every other thing in this book, but I hope you'll be able to recall this one chapter, and that it will have helped you change your professional life for the better.

### Exercise 3–1

**Write on one side of an index card your personal professional goal.** Add the steps needed to achieve it. **Carry the card with you,** and **check it every working day.** Take care to **put in some time on your goal daily,** even if it's only five minutes; make it a habit.

### Who Dictates Your Schedule?

Since we started school, other people have been telling us how we should spend our time:

"Be at this lecture hall at 9 AM."

"Report to that ward for rounds at 7 AM."

"*All surgical residents and fellows to the pathology lab, immediately!*"

We get so used to being ordered around 24 hours a day for 10 or 12 years that it seems only natural, when we're out in practice, to have our office staff, our physician coordinator, or (these days) a computer tell us where to be and what we should be doing every

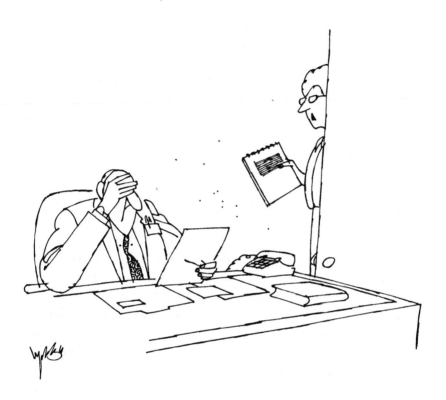

"You have a vendor at one, patients at two, a staff meeting at four, a mock disaster drill at five, and a migraine tonight…"

minute of our working lives. We rush around at top speed trying to keep to their schedule, often falling behind, then scrambling faster to catch up—

*Whoa!*

We're not in training any more. We're mature practitioners, quite capable of self-managing our own time. We need to change our attitude radically here, because *if we don't take back full control of our time, we'll never be free of time pressures and stress.*

> ❝It is wiser to hand over our checkbook to someone else than to hand over our datebook.❞
>
> Jean-Louis Servan-Schreiber[5(p.112)]

Of course we have to delegate some of the detail work of fine-tuning our schedules. About 45% of practitioners do use some kind of computerized scheduling software,[6] and it would be unproductive to waste your time micromanaging your daily appointments and procedures. But you must be the person who decides what your schedule and calendar look like. Only one person can be in charge of something; if it's someone else, it's not you.

### It's Time to Take Back Control of Your Schedule

Someone else (or a computer) dictating our schedule might work to make us more efficient for the short term; but like all solutions imposed on us from outside, it will eventually stop being effective. It reduces us to cogs in the big machine of mass-production medicine. If this assembly-line approach seems efficient to some people, it's only because they haven't yet fully grasped the complex nature of physicians' productivity, which, as we've seen, goes well beyond how many patient visits we can knock out in an hour. It is possible to see more patients in less time, with higher patient satisfaction (as we'll see in Part 4)—but not by becoming an automaton.

And it's more than just our office staff who try to control our schedule; someone is constantly requesting us to do things that we know are a waste of our time, for example:

✦ serve on administrative committees, many of which are inefficient or useless, or both—as in the couplet, "The only committee that gets anything done/Is a committee of one"
✦ attend long, unproductive conferences and meetings
✦ handle extra paperwork, phone calls, audits, surveys, reports, and conferences
✦ handle cases that someone else could handle more competently and more efficiently, and on and on.

As a result, our schedules end up so full that we find the only time we have for our own purposes is the time nobody else wants!

Taking control of your schedule is the first and necessary step toward all the other time management techniques: optimizing, time shifting, flexing, blocking, and the like. Because unless you're in charge, you'll never be able to prune and reshape your workday to fit your unique needs and style of practice. If someone else makes your schedule for you, you'll always feel you're "running behind."

So, starting today—and from here on, every day for the rest of your professional life—**take charge of your own schedule!** Analyze your workday to make sure that you're spending your time doing what makes sense to you, achieving what you wish to achieve.

But first, in order to take charge, you're going to have to **say no to all unreasonable intrusions on your time**.

## The Doctor Who Couldn't Say No

Saying no isn't easy for doctors; we didn't go into this profession to turn down people who ask us for help. Research on medical students shows that the overwhelming reason we chose medicine was the wish to serve others. (Status and income were less popular reasons.) We're so anxious to be of service—and feel so guilty if we're not—that the word "no" often sticks in our throats. Literally.

At an evening seminar for surgeons I asked everyone in the audience to yell "No!" at the top of their lungs, just to get the hang of it. Amazingly, after everyone else in the room roared "No!" one person in the corner said softly but very clearly, "yes." And no matter how many times we shouted "No!" this doctor kept saying, "yes."

"Well, I think our problems here are solved," someone finally observed. "Anytime we're asked to do something unreasonable, we know who to call!"

It was meant as a joke, but that's actually not a bad idea. For example, if someone asks you to serve on a time-wasting committee, say, "No, I can't do it...but why don't you try Dr. Brown? That would be right up his alley. Here's his pager number." Very polite, gets the person off your back quickly, and doesn't sound like a turndown. (Of course, if Dr. Brown is using this same system you have a problem.)

When they suggest that maybe you could do it later, just say, "Look, I don't want to disappoint you by making you think I'm going to be able to do that; I'm not."

A key attitude change for doctors: Saying no is not negative. It won't make your personality sour or turn your aura black. In fact, *saying no is a positive way of prioritizing your own time* more efficiently. Once you realize this, it's easy to keep work off your schedule that doesn't fit your priorities.

And the more you do it, the easier it gets. That's why I always have my seminar audiences shout "No!" over and over. They're a little weak on the first try, but after a few warm-ups they get into it, and the room really rocks.

I make it a point to randomly say no to some perfectly reasonable requests, just to keep my co-workers from taking my availability and general good nature for granted. This habit also keeps my no muscles in good tone, and keeps me consciously in control of my time, so when the pressure is on I can still say clearly, convincingly, and commandingly... *"No!"*

Saying no also gets easier as you get older. One day you wake up and look at yourself in the mirror and realize that you only have *x* days left to get your own life's work done. From that point, you stop suffering fools gladly.

But please, don't put this book down and start running around saying no to everyone you meet. That wouldn't be sensible, and they'll just get angry at you. Use your judgment.

 **Exercise 3–2** Leave off reading for a moment and think of all the other things you might be doing right now: browsing journals, making phone calls, exercising, socializing, whatever. Now say out loud, "No, I'm not doing any of those other things now. I am choosing to read this book, to become more efficient at my practice." Keep saying it for a while, until you can feel that you are the active master of your own time, in this moment.

Savor that feeling.

## Systematically Debride Your Schedule

To take back control of your time, you need to develop another regular habit: schedule debridement. Just as you regularly throw stuff out of your home and your garage (or they'd get so full you'd eventually have to move to a motel), you need to systematically remove all the old, useless, devitalized stuff from your schedule.

Just think for a moment about everyone who's busy right now putting things *on* your schedule: your office and hospital staffs, your patients, your friends, your colleagues, your residents and protégés, pharmaceutical reps, your family, your pets, your indoor plants.

But who have you put in charge of systematically going through your schedule and calendar every day with the express instruction: "Take stuff off"?

Exactly.

Nobody.

And that's the reason your schedule has gotten so crazy.

High-performance corporate CEOs have developed the routine of systematically reviewing their calendars and throwing stuff off, or paying someone a pot of money to do this valuable chore. Otherwise, they'd soon choke on their own schedules. We're also in demand, highly paid, and overscheduled. It's time we adopted the same method.

> ❝[S]ystems normally contain major chunks of useless work....The empowerment comes in giving the workforce the time...to find and remove the waste.❞
>
> Donald Berwick, MD[7(p.622)]

When elected chief of staff for the first time, I found that my secretary had me scheduled to attend almost 20 hours of meetings every week. I immediately had her cancel all of them.

For some weeks, no one missed me at all. Then gradually people started phoning, and I was able to decide on a case-by-case basis whether any given meeting was important enough to attend. Finally, I settled on about five meetings per week, maximum, and was able to get a lot of useful work done for the medical staff in the time I saved.

For the past few years, I've been keeping my administrative activities to a lower level. I've sat on or chaired no more than two medical staff committees—two that are interesting to me, and where I feel I can be productive. But recently I've become department co-chair, so I've just dropped one of those two committees. Because I observe this rule: **Never add anything new to your schedule unless you can eliminate something old.** Doctors have trouble with this, but if you think about it, not following this rule is insane, because your schedule would keep expanding infinitely! In my own case, sticking closely to this rule has kept my calendar from filling up with too many activities, so I can work on my personal professional goal. I only wish that this rule were followed by whoever it is that keeps adding new forms and other paperwork to our load.

 **Exercise 3–3** Take a copy of your monthly schedule to a quiet place where you won't be interrupted. Study it intently, reflecting coolly on what your typical workday is like. Ask these questions about every activity on your schedule:

- Is this still a high priority for me?
- What, if anything, will happen if I do less of this? None at all?
- Can someone else be doing this?
- In five years, will my doing or not doing this matter to anyone?

Then begin systematically crossing out those activities and obligations which don't fit your personal priorities. Inform your office manager of your new procedure for simplifying your schedule.

Repeat prn, but at least every two weeks.

Remember: this is *your* schedule, not anyone else's; you're the only person who can allocate your time wisely. Be cruel to be kind...to yourself. Once you make the first cut, it will get easier. If you've cut that one wasted hour, why not also cut those other two? Get your pen slashing, really enjoy the rhythm. If you can't cut 10% of your schedule, maybe you're not being ruthless enough. If you need ideas about what to cut, look at the "dirty dozen" list in Chapter 4.

Repeat this whole process every couple of weeks, because useless stuff accumulates on your schedule every day, like dust bunnies under your bed.

Don't worry that you'll end up with idle time on your hands. Soon enough, other people will rush in with new demands on your time. And read on for suggestions about replacing the garbage time you've just eliminated with productive activities.

When you succeed in taking back your schedule, you can feel during every moment of the workday that you're doing what you want to do, that nothing else is pulling at you, and that you are now in command of your time—not vice versa. You're in control! It's a nice feeling.

As a highly skilled professional, you should never accept anything less.

---

### Notes

1. T. Peters, *Thriving on Chaos* (New York: Harper & Row, 1987), 498.
2. "Professional Groups Report Turnaround in Physician Income," *Mental Health Economics,* June 1997, 4–5.
3. H. Selye, *The Stress of Life* (New York: McGraw-Hill, 1976), 438.
4. S. Winston, *The Organized Executive* (New York: Warner Books, Inc., 1983), 205.
5. J.-L. Servan-Schreiber, *The Art of Time* (London: Bloomsbury, 1989), 112.
6. "Analyzing the Market for Practice Management Software," *Health Data Management,* April 1996, 66.
7. D. Berwick, "A Primer on Leading the Improvement of Systems," *British Medical Journal* 312 (1996): 619–622.

$\blacklozenge$ **4** $\blacklozenge$

# How to Eliminate Time-Wasting Work Habits

You now have a personal professional goal and a daily schedule that's a bit lighter. But you haven't yet touched the biggest hunk of your time: your hours of routine clinical work. In this chapter we'll demonstrate how your productivity gets sabotaged during an average day and give some specific suggestions for eliminating time wasters.

## Pareto and His Principle

If you've read anything on time management, you're probably familiar with Wilfred Pareto. He was a 19th century Swiss economist who looked at how much money everyone in Switzerland made. Pareto found that incomes were not evenly distributed: in fact, 80% of the money went to just 20% of the population.

Then he studied income distributions in other countries, and came up with pretty much the same finding. In all the countries Pareto looked at, 80% of the income went to 20% of the people.

This rule has come to be called the Pareto Principle, or simply the "80/20" rule, and it seems to hold roughly not only for income distribution, but for many other human activities. In business, 80% of a company's sales ordinarily come from 20% of its customers;

80% of movie studio profits come from 20% of films; 80% of health plan expenditures are incurred by 20% of patients, and so forth.[1]

For workers, the Pareto Principle indicates that 80% of our results are produced by 20% of our efforts. This seems counterintuitive at first. Why should 20% of our efforts produce so much, while the other 80% is, by contrast, pretty much wasted on low-productivity activities? Why should some of our hours be golden —and the rest, garbage?

## Pareto and Your Practice

Pareto's rule will make more sense, I think, if we look at it as a derivative of the familiar bell curve (Figure 4–1). If we plot yield versus activities, out at the far right end of the bell curve will be high-yield activities that we don't do often, but are extremely productive.

Whatever the exact percentages, we can accept this general principle: For any activity we do over time, most of our productiv-

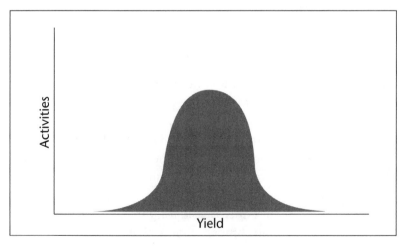

**Figure 4–1** Bell curve of activities and yield.

ity tends to occur during a relatively small segment of the total, when we are super-efficient. Not only is our efficiency high during those times, but we feel almost no sense of friction or excess effort, and our psychological stress level is optimal. We call this state of highly productive absorption in an activity being "in the flow"; for musicians it's "in the groove"; for athletes, "in the zone." Physicians sometimes will say after a particularly smooth and productive day, "I was really doccin' today."

Discussing this point, one enthusiastic specialist at a medical staff seminar blurted, "Yeah, I have some days when I feel so good about my work, I would do it for free!" The hospital medical director, sitting in the back of the room and always alert to a cost-cutting opportunity, called out, *"Get that doctor's name!"*

We all have some hours or days when we're aware of getting a lot accomplished, making a sort of effortless effort, clicking steadily through our clinical routines with an unbroken rhythm. We feel like Gene Kelly at the beginning of *An American in Paris*— that scene where he transforms making his bed and getting his breakfast into a graceful, efficient dance. (A pediatrician told me that her mentor taught her how to perform physical examinations on young children as a dance, smoothly and effortlessly.)

Such work has a distinctive texture:

✦ We don't feel overwhelmed, but we don't feel bored.
✦ We're not being interrupted.
✦ We're optimally "in sync" biologically and psychologically with the work flow.
✦ Our attention is fully absorbed in what we're doing.
✦ Our team is working like clockwork, friction free.

Sounds great. But can we actually make every day "just doccin'"—smooth and highly efficient, so we feel like we're dancing instead of dragging?

The short answer is, Why not?

## Turn Garbage into Gold

Pareto also discovered (though it's rarely mentioned) that the 80:20 ratio is flexible. Look at the bell curve again. What happens if we systematically shift our use of time so that we make the unproductive activities less frequent, and the more productive ones more frequent? The whole curve would then shift to the right, producing a net increase in our productivity.

The economist John Maynard Keynes exemplified the 80/20 rule in his workday. He is said to have labored extremely productively for two hours every day. He would then take the rest of the day off, visiting art galleries, the ballet, and so forth.

If you think about it, you'll notice that each golden hour of super-efficient work is 16 times as productive as one of those garbage hours (because the ratios of input time to output are 4:1 and 1:4, respectively, and $4 \times 4 = 16$). *Logically, then, if we can convert even one of those garbage hours that we're wasting every day into a very efficient hour, we'll get a huge jump in our total productivity.*

Easily said—but how to do it?

## Time-Shifting Increases Your Efficiency

After a productivity seminar, an orthopedic surgeon from Nebraska told me she did procedures and saw patients for three days every week, then spent a full two days doing paperwork. Plainly, every hour of paperwork she could eliminate—and devote to doing more procedures—would increase her productivity for that hour by several times, since doing paperwork was a waste of her skills. We talked about smarter computerization, learning touch-typing, hiring and training some specialized clerical help, even changing her practice so she would have a less onerous paperwork load (she was doing a lot of workers' comp cases). She went home determined to start finding ways of converting paperwork hours into procedure hours.

Maybe your situation is not as clear-cut as the orthopedic surgeon's, but some careful self-analysis will definitely turn up opportunities to **convert less efficient and less satisfying garbage time into golden time**. Study your schedule, and think about it: Start by asking, "What am I doing during the garbage hours? What are my principal time wasters during an average day?"

Every physician group at every seminar I've ever given has had pretty much the same list of time wasters, because we all do pretty much the same general types of tasks. You may be more efficient at minimizing some of the items on this list, but you'll probably agree that some of these things can waste significant chunks of your time and effort:

## The "Dirty Dozen": Major Time Wasters

1. Paperwork
2. Interruptions
3. Re-work (including repairing others' unsatisfactory work)
4. Unnecessary work (overdoing) and omissions (underdoing)
5. Insufficient personal skill or knowledge
6. Clinical errors
7. Missing or misplaced patient information
8. Phone calls
9. Administrative duties and useless meetings
10. Friction, misunderstandings, etc. with others on your team
11. Down time (commuting, waiting for people, unavailable OR, computer or other equipment failure, etc.)
12. Low energy, boredom, depression

These 12 time wasters are so pervasive in every physician's practice that we're going to give specific suggestions for systematically rooting out every one of them.

Here are some suggested remedies for the biggest time killers:

## Don't Under-Do a Task

If you look around your desk right now you'll probably find a number of unfinished projects. These are things you started to work on with high hopes, but just couldn't finish—so they lie around gathering dust, coffee rings, and donut crumbs.

A good rule to adopt right now is: **Don't start any project that you won't finish.**

I'm amazed at how much time and effort I personally save these days just by observing this one rule. My wife says it's because I'm a Gemini, but I have no trouble thinking up a hundred different things I'd like to accomplish: designing research projects, reading review articles and books, taking courses, listening to audiotapes, giving grand rounds on some interesting cases, learning new computer programs, doing a regular physical workout, etc., etc. As a result, my office (and my life) used to be littered with half-done, abandoned projects.

Time study experts say that we may waste 5% to 10% of our time working on things we never finish—and we don't get any credit for what we start, only for what we finish.

There was a famous explorer named Stanley (the one who found Livingstone in the African jungle and greeted him, "Dr. Livingstone, I presume?"). Stanley had a good motto: **Finish just one thing every day.**

We could adopt his motto and immediately see our productivity shoot up, because not a day would pass when we wouldn't finish something. I've found that looking around for half-done projects to finish—and not starting anything new that I probably won't be able to complete—has increased the amount I actually produce.

Also, having all those half-done jobs rankling in the back of your brain draws off some of your concentration and mental energy, even if you're not conscious of it. Not to speak of the fact that your workspace gets cluttered and your morale gets pulled down every time you look at your stacks of unfinished stuff.

**Exercise 4–1** Find all the unfinished projects around your office. Sort them into two piles: those you can finish quickly (and still want to finish), and those you probably will never finish (or could care less about). Throw away the second pile.

Start working on the easiest (or most interesting) project in the remaining pile, and stay at it until it's finished. Repeat until the pile is gone.

Before you take on any new project, ask yourself, "Will I ever finish this?" Be honest. Don't start any new project you probably won't finish. Use the time you save to finish your other projects, especially those relating to your professional goal.

A surgery professor asked me after a seminar how to choose among several unfinished clinical research projects—which should he complete first? I had no idea, but I suggested he might decide on the basis of his own psychology. Was he the sort of person who liked to get some closure right away? Then he might choose the shortest project. Or was there one project that especially stimulated his enthusiasm? Or was there one that needed to be rushed more than the others? In other words, as with most questions, he could decide this one on its merits—but he definitely should pick one project and finish it, and dispose of all his unfinished projects before he started any new ones.

One small caveat: Many of us docs are perfectionists, so we have to be careful not to be overly strict with this rule. Don't punish yourself by compulsively finishing tasks that you hate; finish what you really want to finish, and what you'll enjoy having accomplished.

Which brings us to the next suggestion.

## Don't Overdo a Task

Besides not starting things we won't finish, or under-working, we tend to overwork at things that are already done. If you've done as much as you can on a patient's case, don't keep fiddling with it. Some of the worst medicine I've ever practiced happened because I didn't know when to quit and call in someone else. This is such a useful principle, and applies to so much of our clinical work, that we need to look at it more closely.

For example, in Figure 4–2 you'll recognize the familiar S curve of drug dose and effect. When you first give certain drugs, nothing much happens for a while (A), because the drug has to build up in the serum or plasma. But when it reaches a certain minimum level—the threshold (Thresh) for that drug in that patient—a lot starts to happen; in this part of the curve (B), small increments in the drug dose can give you a lot of bang for your buck.

Then, if you keep giving more and more drug, the effect levels off, and after a certain point you can raise the dose all you want and it makes little difference—you've reached the saturation

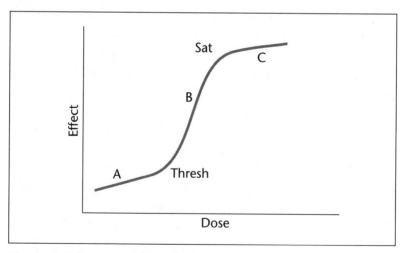

**Figure 4–2** S-curve of drug dose and effect.

point (Sat) of maximum effect for that particular drug in that patient (C), and not much more is going to happen (except more side effects and toxicity).

Besides drug dose and effect, the ratio of effort (and other inputs) to output tends to follow this same curve. For instance, when we take a medical history, after asking a certain number of questions in a patient interview, we start to get fewer positive answers. We can keep asking more questions, but our efficiency drops off.

It is also common experience that in working up a clinical case, we take a while to get going as we start from ground zero and get the initial history, exams, tests, etc. (A in the figure). Then, as our information accumulates and we begin to see patterns of possible diagnoses and treatments more clearly, our work begins to move faster in the gold zone (B).

However, if we keep at it too long, we can reach a point of diminishing returns, and our case just gets overwrought without much more benefit accruing (C). Medical students typically overdo when they're learning how to work up a patient—they may actually have all the information they need for a diagnosis, but they keep on doing more (and less relevant) tests and examinations.

So there's a saturation point for each of our clinical tasks, beyond which we can keep working, but our efficiency will go down—in short, we may be wasting time or resources.

## Working in the Gold Zone

The S curve also describes how we all intuitively practice medicine. None of us wants to work below the threshold, where we're doing less than what is clearly necessary for a patient, nor do we want to work above the saturation point, where we're ordering tests and procedures that are clearly excessive. All of us want to work as much as possible in the gold zone.

We can also think of this curve as representing a continuum of care for our patients. The gold zone could be re-labeled "appropriate care." "Inappropriate care" would be doing either too little (maybe trying to save some money), or too much (wasting resources).[2]

> For all professionals, eliminating time wasted on redundant activities is the quickest way to increase productivity.

Obviously, these days we're all highly motivated to work in the gold zone, where the patient gets optimal care, and unnecessary care (and expense) is avoided. The hot arguments are usually about how far down the slope toward the threshold of being unsafe some payer wants us to work, to save money.

If you understand this curve, and where you're working along it in a given case, you may be able to make more logical decisions about efficient inputs of time, effort, and resources versus safety. You may also win more arguments with payers about whether a certain level of inputs is appropriate to a given case.

Sometimes we overdo an individual case because we're feeling uncomfortable or inadequate. I'm sure you've seen practitioners who keep trying to do more and more in a case that isn't going too well under their care; they can't bring themselves to graciously hand the patient off to a colleague for a second opinion. We all do this occasionally, and it's worthwhile to ask ourselves in such situations whether our ego is keeping us overinvolved.

Some good things that happen to us when we work in the gold zone of optimum effort:

✦ We feel in control—of the case, and of the available resources.

✦ We're most efficiently using our talents, skills, and knowledge.

✦ The challenges closely match our abilities, so we work "in the flow" without much friction or conscious effort.

✦ We feel we're helping, fighting—and winning!

This optimum match of resources to tasks can be a peak experience for physicians, so try to achieve it every day. Being careful not to overdo nor under-do can increase your productivity, your safety, and your satisfaction.

## Learning in the Gold Zone

How many times do you have to do a procedure before you become really excellent at it?

Obviously, a lot more than once—"See one, do one, teach one" is more usually "See one, screw two, do one." In fact, the actual number of repetitions varies according to the complexity of the procedure and the talent of the practitioner.

As an example, for laparoscopic hernia repairs, practitioner excellence seems to develop somewhere between the 50th and 200th procedure.[3] Much below those numbers, you're more likely to be in the (A) section of the learning curve. For cardiologists, doing fewer than 75 angioplasties annually seems to be associated with less excellent outcomes.[4]

These data imply two things: First, if you've done only 25 of either of these procedures, don't be surprised if you're still getting some problematic outcomes. Second, surgeons and invasive cardiologists doubtless want to improve the learning curve so that mastery comes earlier and with less variation. (In Part 3, we'll look at some fast ways of learning a new procedure.)

## Is Your Career in the Gold Zone?

Last, you can use the S curve to understand where you stand in your career.

When we start out in a field, at first we're not very efficient (A), and we have to learn a certain amount to become quick and confident at the work. However, if we then keep working for years or decades in that one field, we may find that we reach a saturation point. One day we realize that the work we're doing no longer challenges us; it's too routine, we're not stimulated, and we're not learning very much (C).

This happened to me after about 12 years of practicing one particular subspecialty. After doing the same thing every day for so long, I found myself feeling stale and restless; sometimes I was just going through the motions. My thoughts started running to other things during the workday, and I even began to fantasize about early retirement.

Then one summer, by a happy fluke, I found myself working temporarily in a university department of geriatric psychiatry, a subspecialty I had not seriously considered. The heavy medical emphasis jump-started a neglected part of my brain; I found I was enjoying the challenge. When an opportunity came to change subspecialties, I grabbed it; I've never looked back.

Performance experts claim that your personal productivity can go up as much as 40% if you and your working environment are a good "fit." If, to achieve this fit, you need to consider a mid-career correction, then so be it. Probably because of the rapidity of knowledge dissemination and the intensity of clinical experience, some practitioners these days may find themselves thinking about a change after about seven to ten years in one specialty. I've worked with several residents who changed their specialties after age 50. They all said it was the right decision—for them.

 **Exercise 4–2** Take one full minute to review where you are on the S curve of your own career. Are you still enthusiastic about your work? Learning something new daily? Feeling stimulated and interested much of the time?

If not, what changes can you make to improve your situation? Can you start now?

We may overwork at a task when we can't control our work environment. One Christmas Eve afternoon I overheard a local urologist trying to dictate a case summary in the nurses' station. He would start, get interrupted, start again, get interrupted again, etc. This went on for two painful hours.

No case summary needs to take two hours—especially not on Christmas Eve. Which brings us to one of our biggest time wasters.

## Eliminate Most Interruptions

Recently one seminar attendee wrote me, "I'm saving six hours per week by following the commandments."

Well, these are not commandments, they're just suggestions based on what other practitioners have found works for them.

Except for this one, which *is* a commandment: **Don't allow any unreasonable interruptions while you're working!**

*Warning! Note these exceptions:* Emergencies (actual and potential) and correcting errors you may have made.

It's inherent in the complexity and unpredictability of clinical work that there will be interruptions—they just shouldn't happen to us.

But why should it be the *physician* who's never interrupted? What about our nursing staff? Don't they have the same rights? (In fact, an article in the *American Journal of Nursing* warned nurses also not to allow interruptions—especially while they're passing meds. This makes good sense.[5])

In general, however, here's why we should be allowed to work without interruption: Nurses and office staff, by necessity, are already doing what the time study people call "interrupted work": one minute they're answering patient requests, next they're checking a chart, then they're preparing a treatment, then they're making a note or answering a phone call. By the nature of their job description, nurses can rarely keep at one task for very long without legitimate interruptions.

But for the patient's sake, *someone on the team has to be able to apply their brain continuously to the thorny task of solving complex clinical problems, one-pointedly following involved trains of thought over extended periods of uninterrupted concentration.*

That person has to be *you*.

No one else can do it as well. So **insist on uninterrupted time to do your work**. You'll have to manage this one yourself—others cannot fully appreciate your need for continuous concentration. But look how important this is.

### INTERRUPTIONS ARE COSTING YOU 20 HOURS WEEKLY

Studies show that workers in an average office are interrupted every six minutes. On a busy hospital floor or in the clinic, the rate is higher. It seems we're constantly getting called and paged out of rounds, conferences, patient interviews, and periods of intense thought.

Worse, research shows that it actually takes about four minutes to get back up to full speed after an interruption. So if we're getting interrupted every six minutes, and it takes us four minutes to get back up to our former level of efficiency—no wonder we're not getting much done!

Most physicians report to us that they get interrupted about three times during a standard 15-minute patient visit. That doesn't sound too bad, but given the four-minute recovery period, that adds up to 20 hours per week of disrupted, low-productivity work if we allow interruptions.

And if you're interrupted while working with your team or with a patient, then their time is also being wasted during the interruptions, *multiplying the lost time by two, five, or ten times*. The next time you're on rounds and get interrupted, just watch everyone standing around doing nothing for the length of the interruption, and realize how much time is being wasted. After that, I don't think you'll let anyone interrupt.

Studies of why we're being interrupted in the first place give us more reason to abolish interruptions: Most of the time, for instance, incoming phone calls actually turn out to be less important than the work they interrupt.[6]

### WHEN COLLEAGUES INTERRUPT

"But I need those interruptions!" complained a young internist last year. "Those calls are sometimes referrals from other docs, and I need referrals." Recently, however, this physician told me she has now stopped taking most calls while she's working at something else. Weighing the lost productivity caused by interruptions against the risk of losing the odd referral, she has decided to work straight through. She figures she makes up in effectiveness and accuracy what she may occasionally lose by not taking calls—and that she probably gets more referrals now because she can work in a concentrated way to get better outcomes. She has made sure her office staff recognize referral calls and get them to her attention quickly when she has a break.

Interruptions will shatter your work rhythms. Scoping a colon isn't exactly doing the rumba, but all of our medical work has subtle but definite rhythms that are complex and can be easily disrupted. Rhythms make work easier, smoother, faster. If you're a surgeon you probably play your favorite music in the OR, and if you work out, you know that the right cassette can make that stairstepping go much more quickly. On the other hand, constantly losing and having to recover our work rhythms—because we're interrupted—subtly drains energy and pushes up our stress.

Worst of all, *interruptions are a major cause of clinical errors.* For this reason alone, we need to get rid of them.

I hope you're now convinced that you need to eliminate interruptions from your work.

(Besides the two exceptions mentioned above, if you need to make other exceptions to guarantee safe practice, of course do so. And if you personally prefer to be interrupted while you work, by all means continue your own preferred practice pattern.)

 **Exercise 4–3** Train your staff not to interrupt you except for emergencies, or to correct an error. Take them all aside and explain the reasons for your request. Make sure they understand the exceptions. Tell your office manager about the new policy, and thank everyone profusely when they make the change.

If someone persists in interrupting your work, be firm but not rude: "What you're saying is so important that I want to give it my full attention, so let's get to it when I've finished doing this procedure. Thanks." They'll take the hint.

If it suits your personal working style, try having your staff arrange your work seamlessly, without frequent breaks and pauses. This seems to help some practitioners avoid interruptions by keeping up a steady flow and rhythm. Another helpful habit is to structure your daily staff interactions with a simple query such as, "Anything I need to know?" or "Anything pressing?"—before you start your work. That gives your staff a chance to communicate with you on your own schedule, instead of trying to interrupt you later.

To get a no-interruptions policy to work, you have to set a prestige example yourself. If your staff person is hard at work on something urgent, interrupt her only if your matter truly can't wait. On the other hand, if she's gossiping about her weekend or the scandal in the next office, and you're trying to get real work done, *always* interrupt—politely, of course.

One internist told me, "I'm saving a significant amount of time by not taking calls while I'm working...now I just have to figure out how to get my wife to speak to me again, since I don't take her calls, either." (Actually, I've met his wife, and I'm sure she'll understand.)

## Cut Time Spent in Useless Meetings...

Most doctors don't like meetings, because we recognize intuitively that they're not only an interruption, but usually a waste of our work time.

On this point we differ from executives and managers, who love meetings, and will even boast to each other, "So-and-so gave me a meeting." The difference stems from the fact that as physicians we usually do our work one on one; that's just the nature of our tasks. In contrast, managers are not rewarded for the work they do for individuals, but for how much work they can get groups of other people to do. And one very effective way for managers to get people to do things is to have meetings.

For docs, most meetings are inefficient. Here are some suggestions from busy physicians for cutting down the waste:

1. **Don't go to any meeting unless your secretary has called ahead to confirm it is actually happening.** Studies show that 50% of meetings are canceled, postponed, or moved, or do not follow the announced agenda. For some reason, meetings called by non-physician managers and administrators are canceled more often than physician-led meetings. If a meeting has already been rescheduled once, it's more likely to be canceled a second time (probably for the same reason)—so check extra carefully before you go.
2. How many meetings are you attending just because you're used to going? **Eliminate habit meetings from your schedule.**

3. If there's a meeting you're somewhat interested in, but would rather not attend, **get on the "minutes-only" list**, or have someone get you the handout. You can read the record of what went on in about 1/30th of the time you'd spend in the meeting.
4. If there's a meeting you think might actually be productive, **have someone go in your place**. Better yet, find two other physicians and **form a network** so each of you can attend one-third of the meetings in rotation, representing the other two and keeping them posted on anything important.
5. It's not your job to make a meeting efficient, interesting, and worthwhile. If the chairperson or speaker is not doing his job, **pull out a reprint or your laptop**—or pull your whole self out of the meeting and go work on your personal goal. Don't stand on ceremony. Your time is valuable, and they should realize this.
6. If the meeting is being given by someone to inflate their ego, or **if the meeting has become a ritual, walk**.

### ...to Leave More Time for Useful Meetings

On the other hand, it is crucial to attend certain meetings.

You might not think of it as a meeting, but that little first-thing-in-the-morning stand-up (I sit down) with your staff not only gives everyone a chance to get their first cup of caffeine, it gets the maximum amount of information to everyone in the shortest possible time, smooths out the schedule, and sets your team's rhythm for the rest of the day. Keep it short.

Most physicians agree you need to **get to at least one large educational meeting of your specialty association (or to a university-sponsored update in your field) every year or two**. We'll see later how having up-to-date knowledge makes your use of time much more efficient.

But an association meeting is more than a place to benchmark your clinical knowledge against the state of the art and spot new trends—it's also a chance to hang out with pals and colleagues, get some inspiration, meet new friends, get away from the usual routine for a while and think, hear great speakers, etc. When I give seminars for medical and surgical associations, I'm careful to make my presentations entertaining, inspiring, and information-dense. These meetings usually are a productive way for you to spend your time, but if you're not entirely happy with the content or style of presentations, make sure your association's program committee knows about it. Believe me, they very much want you to come back next year, and they'll listen.

These days it may also be crucial for you to show up at certain administrative meetings, especially if you're in the middle of a push-pull between physicians and non-physicians about health care decisions in your community. **If your presence and voice can make a difference, attend administrative meetings**—it's also time well invested, in the long run.

---

**Notes**

1. J. Sokolov, Interview, *Quality Connection*, Summer 1994, 7.
2. D. Mirvis, "Managed Care, Managing Uncertainty," *Archives of Internal Medicine* 157 (1997): 385–388.
3. L. Kennedy, "Study Explores Causes of Laparoscopic Hernia Repair Failure," *General Surgery and Laparoscopy News*, May 1997, 1–11.
4. E.L. Hannan et al, "Coronary Angioplasty Volume—Outcome Relationships for Hospitals and Cardiologists," *Journal of the American Medical Association* 277, no. 11 (1997): 892–898.
5. N.M. Davis, "Concentrating on Interruptions," *American Journal of Nursing*, March 1994, 14.
6. "Productive Calling," *Success Magazine*, September 1994, 33.

## ✦ 5 ✦

# How to Cut Paperwork, Phone Calls, and Procrastination

Every physician I've talked to agrees that, of all time wasters, the worst is paperwork.

With or without computerized support, the average physician spends 25% of her total workday processing data.[1] The computer was supposed to relieve the paperwork load, but instead, by the law of unintended consequences, it has actually increased the avalanche. If you don't believe there's now more paperwork than ever, just drive over to your local office supply megastore. You'll find on sale at the front of the store (right next to the computers) an entire wall of paper, as big as a railroad freight car—all waiting to be filled out.

## Transitioning to Computers

As this is being written, our profession is definitely moving toward fully computerized clinical information systems. If you're already doing some of your clinical work on a keyboard, you know that a good electronic system can increase your speed on information-intensive tasks—by as much as 30%, some physicians have told me. A recent study of physicians using a computer-based records system confirmed a 13% increase in patient visits.[2]

So why have only about one in 20 offices switched to the paperless chart?[3] The answers I hear most often are: "My operation is too small to justify it," "The hardware and software are too expensive," "It takes too much training, maintenance, and updating," and, "I'm definitely looking into it for the future."

Electronic clinical information systems seem to be most popular in larger organizations (the military and large HMOs, e.g.) which service a lot of patients in huge, spread-out facilities where paper would be a nightmare, and where big investment is possible. Physicians who are happiest with their systems report that they got guidance and support from someone with a similar practice who already had a system; that previous PC background helps, but is not crucial; and that getting a day or so of training on the system is important.

Future systems promise to go far beyond replacing our paper charts: entire medical textbooks, MEDLINE, clinical decision support software, real-time video consultation, etc., will all be available on a small screen near you (more on using your PC for clinical decision making in Part 3).

However, don't look for computers to actually reduce the amount of annoying paperwork—hard copy or electronic—for you to do. When I've pinned down administrators of facilities that are computerized, they admit that data processing is still a major chore in spite of all the new gadgets for handling it.

So paperwork isn't going away, and we all have to learn how to do it more efficiently, if we're going to be more productive. Fortunately, the general principles for handling paperwork as painlessly as possible are essentially the same, whether or not you're computerized.

## With Paperwork, Less Is Much Better

Paperwork by itself has no value in producing good clinical outcomes. The exceptions are carefully thought out notes or evaluations; writing or dictating one of these may help you organize and clarify a complex case. But in general, the more quickly and efficiently we get through this chore, the better. The point is to cut down time spent on paperwork as much as feasible, while (1) maintaining our clinical records at the necessary optimum level for our own and others' future use, and (2) keeping up our reimbursements.

In fact, for both these purposes, less is usually more, since both payers and clinicians prefer terse, crisp clinical communication. This sounds obvious—but I'm amazed at how many docs still turn out lengthy, woolly reports. Last week I asked a cardiologist for his recommendation on a patient, so I could get a procedure authorized. Yesterday I received his two-page consult—with lots of details, but without the simple recommendation I needed, and which I had clearly requested. Now I have to call him again and ask him to do it over. He's wasted his time—and mine.

Most successful physicians we've spoken with agree that you can cut your total paperwork time by 5% to 20%—but you have to **use aggressive methods of paperwork reduction,** and you have to **be assertive and disciplined, and stick to it religiously**. Paperwork is a blobby monster that can infiltrate your whole workday unless you go after it. If you find yourself staying after hours to catch up on paperwork, stop doing that. Instead, declare your private war on paperwork now—so you can have some peace.

## The PEACE System

The system that follows is a synthesis of several generally similar paperwork reduction systems used by busy physicians. As with all the other suggestions in this book, you'll need to decide whether using it makes sense for your style of practice, then try it out and customize it for your own situation.

And please do write us if you come up with a better system.

The PEACE System for Paperwork Reduction
P = Prioritize (and do quick, urgent stuff right now)
E = Eliminate (at least 1/2 of your incoming papers)
A = Analyze (what's left, for minimal required input)
C = Complete (touch twice)
E = Edit (cut excess words—then cut more)

## Before You Start

First you'll need some equipment. Stop at an office supply superstore tonight and **buy a huge wastebasket for your office**. It can be as stylish as you want, as long as it's industrial size, *at least 20 gallons*. Paperwork reduction is serious stuff, and the right equipment can save you many hours of wasted time. (If having a really huge wastebasket in your office embarrasses you, get two that are semi-huge.)

Install the enormous wastebasket(s) in your main work area, and make sure there are equally big wastebaskets in any other places where you ordinarily do paperwork.

You'll find that enormous gaping basket just *sucks* the papers right out of your hands. Never again will you have to keep useless papers floating around because your wastebasket is full. It's like putting giant air intakes and exhausts on a car: Your speed and efficiency go up with a mighty *whoosh*.

Now you're equipped to start doing the dreaded daily paperwork, following the PEACE acronym.

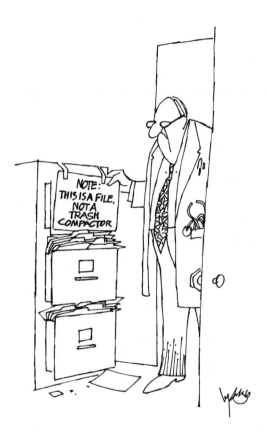

## P (Prioritize) and E (Eliminate)

To prioritize, you first need to triage as much paper out of your in-trays (or electronic documents out of your files) as you possibly can. If you can train someone on your staff to do most of your triaging for you, even better. But no matter how well they do the job, you'll still have to make a final cut.

Assume that the vast majority of paper that comes to you (1) was not meant for you, and should go to someone else; (2) was never meant for anyone, and is pure garbage; or (3) was meant for you, but is a mistake, because you really don't want or need it, so you're probably not going to read it or act on it.

Immediately find, readdress, and dump all the (1) stuff directly into someone else's tray (or put it in the out-tray, or clip and e-mail it), and dump all the (2) and (3) stuff directly into your mega-basket (or electronic trash bin). Be quick, be cruel, be decisive, don't ever look back. This is war.

Among all the junk, you'll find (and save) some important items: patient data and reports and other clinical information, as well as forms you have to fill out to get paid. But believe me, in this age of superfast word processors and high-speed printers, modems, and copying machines, it's so easy to send out useless stuff that most of the paper we all get is just junk. If you've already cut out useless meetings, time-wasting administrative committees, projects you're never going to finish, etc., you won't receive as much worthless paper.

If you find in your pile something that is actually urgent, that's a mistake. Urgent stuff and anything that needs only a second or two to finish (a signature, scrip, brief written question, etc.) should not be in your paper pile at all; someone should have posted it on a "Do Now" clipboard between your examining rooms—or otherwise brought it to your attention—so you can catch it on the fly.

## A (Analyze) and C (Complete)

After dumping or re-routing all the junk, and finishing the brief, time-critical stuff in your clipboards at first touch, you'll still have some papers left. These are not pressing, but they do need to be read and acted on by someone, so analyze them with a view toward getting rid of them quickly:

✦ Can you possibly delegate this to someone else? Can someone just copy a previous completed document, or can you just re-edit a previous form, etc.?

✦ Can this wait until you get a reminder? Should it wait because it's too early, and you might have to re-do later?

✦ Can you quickly train someone else to do this—and have these re-routed to that person from now on?

✦ If it's important, but too long and wordy to read quickly, can you get the crucial facts in summary form, via phone or e-mail, etc.?

✦ If the person on the other end is using an algorithm (standard practice for MCOs), can you get hold of their algorithm and use it to speed your work (and your approval rate)?

✦ Can you get informally trained by a colleague or co-worker in how to do these forms more quickly?

✦ Is this a frequently used form that should be on someone's computer (preferably, someone else's)? Can it be completely automated on a system (Stratford, e.g.)?

✦ Can you create a formula, template, or plug-in response for this type of document, and use it from now on to save time and effort?

We physicians are a little less comfortable than other professionals with using form letters and prompts, which is too bad, because they really can speed up our paperwork and save enormous amounts of wheel-reinventing.

My middle daughter is a newly minted attorney, and a few months back I told her I was having problems with a local trades-man, who had installed an overhead door on my garage that didn't work. I told her, "I've called him several times, but he won't come out and fix it, and he won't refund what I paid him so I can hire someone else. Could you compose a threatening letter I can send him, to get him to fix it?"

"Compose a threatening letter?" my daughter the lawyer said incredulously. "I don't have to *compose* a threatening letter. We have *form* threatening letters!"

If lawyers can use form threatening letters, then we should cer-tainly not stand on ceremony, when we could be using formulas to speed up many of our communications. Any letter or report we particularly admire for its crispness and organization can be saved as a template, or we can get formulas from outside sources (your malpractice insurer has some excellent form letters you can use when dismissing a patient, etc.). All your form letters and re-ports belong in a folder that never leaves your desk (or wherever you usually dictate), or on your hard drive or diskettes.

This is not to say you should copy form letters slavishly. Physi-cians have told me they don't like getting obvious form letters or reports from other practitioners. But you can use the form as a prompt to speed your work, to make sure you've included every-thing crucial, thus avoiding re-do's, etc.

Incidentally, the form threatening letter worked, and the fellow fixed my garage door.

Analyze all your paperwork to establish the absolute minimum needed to satisfy the person on the other end (your intended audi-ence). This is especially useful when filling out insurance forms. Sometimes we pile on the clinical information in the pious hope that (1) this will increase our capture rate for reimbursements, (2) a clinician is at the other end, and (3) somebody besides us actu-ally gives a damn about how and what we write. Usually, none of these things are true. Putting down exactly what's asked for in a terse, formulaic way saves time and usually works better (because they're using formulas, too).

In fact, you can shoot yourself in the foot by saying too much on insurance forms (this is also true on the telephone). The person at the other end may have a list of "10 Ways to Say No" in front of them, and the more you write or talk, the more likely you are to trip one of these.[4] Try spending a few minutes on the phone or over coffee with someone knowledgeable finding out the few magic words needed to ensure certain reimbursements, and skip all the rest.

Don't assume that you're the best person to complete a given piece of paperwork, unless you really are fast and good at handling it, and it's the most effective use of your time. Use the general principle that whoever on your team is best at doing something should be doing it—no standing on ceremony or titles. So what if they don't do it as perfectly as you would—at least it's done.

If you're hand-writing anything—a note, order, scrip, draft, etc.—taking a few extra seconds to make it legible prevents errors, re-do's, and callbacks. Scribbling fast might seem to save time, but studies show we physicians get an incredibly high rate of callbacks for our illegible writing. If a word is one you don't habitually use, or if it could be confused with a similar word, print it. If you're computerized, be aware that keyboarding errors occur at the rate of about one per page, so check for these. If you want to speed up, try a self-tutoring touch-typing program on CD-ROM; some of them are fun.

## E (Edit)

After you've dumped, re-routed, delegated, minimized, form-lettered, and formulized everything you can, there might still be a tiny bit of paperwork left for you actually to do. Complete this without further ado, being as systematic as you can about touching each piece only once more, so you don't waste time sifting and re-sifting old papers.

And whatever you write, whether it's a history, a letter, a report, a chart note, a summary, a consult, or whatever—please edit.

Ernest Hemingway, that master of 20th century prose, was famous for being able to pack a tremendous impact into few words. When someone asked him how he learned to do this, he said that as a cub reporter he had to telegraph his news stories home, at 75 cents a word (equal to about $10 a word now). At those prices, Hemingway learned how to edit his writing into short, muscular sentences.

Our words are just as expensive as Hemingway's. By the time we've stopped whatever else we might be doing to dictate, write, or word process; check over; rewrite (if necessary); and by the time our secretary has word processed, checked, sent, and filed our stuff—and by the time someone on the other end has actually read it through—a lot of money and effort have been spent. Shorter saves time at both ends, so shorten and sharpen everything you write.

Forget *woolly*; think *crisp*.

### How to Cut Phone Time

The telephone was the last word in efficiency 100 years ago, and even today we couldn't practice without it. But like most wonderful inventions, it has turned out to be a mixed blessing. Now that we can also use fax, voicemail, e-mail, etc., we need to **be more careful about using the (voice) telephone**, to avoid wasted time, decreased productivity—and general annoyance.

If you phone a *colleague* during the working day, you have only one chance in four of reaching him on the first try.[5] Since you're more likely to end up talking to his voicemail, it makes sense to leave the most complete and effective message you can, with clear questions that he can answer on your voicemail, if necessary. Lots of clinical business can be done machine-to-machine once you get past thinking of such electronic conversations as telephone tag. But getting a machine when you want a human is frustrating—so do be careful never to leave an abusive or curt message; people don't appreciate hate-voicemail!

Also, *health plan utilization reviewers* will make an ugly note in your dossier if you lose your temper or are uncooperative with them on the phone.[6] It may help to keep in mind that the person you're blowing on is just a messenger, not the root cause of your frustration.

Our office and hospital *nursing staffs* probably phone us more than anyone else, yet docs are taught little or nothing about optimizing these contacts. Surprising fact: Nurses report on surveys that calling a physician is one of the most stressful things they have to do (and they do a lot of stressful things), because so many of us are routinely curt, rude, and cruel when called with even routine requests.[7]

So think about these suggestions, and try to keep them in mind the next time you get called:

✦ Since it's so stressful for them, by the time your nurses do phone you, it usually seems pretty urgent to them, and blowing up—or just hanging up—means you'll probably miss getting some crucial information, or at best a chance to be supportive to a worried co-worker. Sometimes they have to cover their rear ends, too, just as we do.

✦ Realize that while it may be your tenth call that night, it's probably her first, so it makes no sense to take out the other nine on her.

✦ Mumble some pleasantries for a few moments to give yourself time to wake up and become alert before you try to deal with the problem; it could save you having to call back again a few minutes later when your mind is clearer.

✦ Having her repeat your verbal orders ("hearback") is usually required practice, and can save another call later—or an error; it also gives you another chance to review what you've ordered.

✦ If you write your orders and scrips more legibly (or print) you can save time on the phone: 20% of handwritten orders are so illegible that they require a phone call to clarify them. Some docs make it a religion to read out complex orders to a nurse before they leave, eliminating these calls.

✦ And even if you're not feeling too grateful for the phone call, say, "Thank you for calling me" at the end, anyway. It's the rare physician who can be civil at 3 AM, and you'll endear yourself to that nurse forever.

Up to 30% of all physician–*patient* contacts are over the phone, so it's too bad there's not more research and training in how to be efficient in this type of interaction.[8]

You probably stack up follow-up messages from patients and knock them off quickly (or delegate them), since these usually require only reassurance or clarification of instructions. It's more important during this type of phone call to be strong, firm, and cheerful than it is to give a lot of details; research shows that over the phone, the tone of your voice is key, so being positive and energetic can cut down on the time you spend talking, and give better results.

To cut down on the number of follow-up calls from patients, nothing works as well as thorough face-to-face discussions and education in the first place (some or most of which you can delegate, thereby saving you time in two ways).

If you haven't seen them recently, and if you discuss their symptoms on the phone, patients will end up coming in to see you about 60% of the time anyway. Some patients won't tell you certain key facts in their history on the phone, and you obviously can't see, touch, or otherwise examine them efficiently ("How big is the cut? Four centimeters?" etc.). Studies show that patient phone calls require 3 to 15 minutes (average, about 6), so you need to decide if it's more efficient all around just to have callers come in for a short visit, and save the phone time for more productive activities.[9]

If you want to delegate patient phone calls (especially off hours), and you work in a large group (more than ten docs), training one talented nurse to do this job can make sense. If you don't want to tie up your office staff, there are firms you can hire to do this service for you.

However, there's not much evidence that telephone triaging cuts down on visits, since about 40% of triaged patients end up seeing a doc within a few hours. Telephone triage nurses often just use printed or computerized protocols, which isn't the same as actually knowing the patient; in fact, relying on protocols sometimes generates more work and referrals.

## E-Mail and the Humble Fax

As more docs get wired to intranets and the Internet, e-mail is becoming an efficient way to stay in contact with other professionals. But be aware that you (and they) need to check e-mail every day; a lot of physicians don't—thereby pretty much defeating the whole purpose.

People try to warm up their e-mail with little sideways smiley faces :-), but it can't compare with actually talking to another human being. If you work in a big organization, be aware that your e-mail might be monitored, and could end up being posted somewhere embarrassing. External e-mail isn't too reliable—9% of it never arrives; if you need to be sure, use fax or regular mail (99.9% of first class mail gets there—eventually).[10]

A young practitioner working in one of our high-tech counties who lists her e-mail address in her Yellow Pages ad has gotten some new-patient visits this way, but very few. Some docs do keep in touch with patients this way, but because of its unreliability and unpredictable time lags, e-mail is not appropriate for patients who may be having an emergency.

While everyone raves about computer networking and e-mail, a little low-rent gadget on the back shelf goes on churning out important work, completely unnoticed: the fax. Computer snobs stick their noses up at the technology, which dates from the Civil War, and call faxes "transitional," meaning they'll disappear soon; they've been saying this for ten years, and there are now more fax machines than ever (they far outnumber computers). Faxes cost one-fifth of what a computer does, they almost never need expensive updating of their hardware or software, and they're so absurdly simple to use that I've never found one single book about using faxes. The newer faxes will also copy; scan; print; send to multiple addresses; work at night while you sleep; store documents; and send x-rays, EKGs, drawings, reprints, lunch orders, etc. Of course, they're also voice phones.

So as you go through your day of juggling forms, data, and correspondence, look for more ways you can use fax machines to speed up your work; everyone has one, and you don't need a guru to show you how to use them. If your office fax is ancient, consider replacing it with one of the newer multi-use gadgets; you can keep the old one at home—it'll never wear out.

## The Case Against Procrastination

I've been surprised over the years at how many otherwise very productive physicians complain about being procrastinators. Like most humans, we docs tend to do first the things we like, find easy, or that other people ask us to do—and put off the rest.

But whatever we put off doing usually rankles in the back of our brain, subtly sapping our energy and increasing our stress.

By the time you do get to what you've put off, your energy and alertness are lower, and you may have to rush to meet a deadline; both conditions set you up for errors, and for needless stress.

Most galling of all, procrastination is a total fraud. Think about it: The whole point of saying, "I'll do it later" is not having to do something unpleasant (or difficult) now.

The fraud is, that when you finally do the thing you put off, you always have to do it now anyway—i.e., in real time. So the whole thing is a delusion—and you should **eliminate unneeded procrastination**.

What helps, if you're a habitual procrastinator?

✦ Blocking and chipping (see Chapter 6), because you can do things more easily either in smaller bites or all in a row so you build momentum

✦ "Just doing it"—i.e., forcing your mind (which can be stubborn) to action, because procrastination is basically a habit that you can break by never doing it

✦ Working in a team (they'll definitely make you do it now)

✦ Announcing publicly you're going to do something by such and such time

✦ Getting more training in a procedure that you find yourself dreading and/or putting off doing (doctors as a group tend to put off adopting new drugs and procedures)

✦ Remembering what a racket the whole procrastination thing is, and getting mad enough to just do it.

## When to Procrastinate

But in some situations, you should always procrastinate.

Naturally, **procrastinate on those chores (especially paperwork) that you know you'll have to re-do later**. It still surprises me how many docs dictate discharge summaries, e.g., too early—and then have to do them over.

**Procrastinate if a friend requests you to do something you don't want to do,** but you can't say no without destroying the relationship: "I can't write that work excuse for you right now, but I'll try to get to it…catch me later." Keep procrastinating, and even if you never say no outright, they'll get the idea, and look elsewhere. (This also works for people who want to borrow money.)

This suggestion could save your career someday: **Always procrastinate if you're teed off about something and about to take strong action.** "A cut with a scalpel will heal, but a cut with the tongue, never." Being openly at war with a co-worker can make your days (and theirs) really sour, stressful, and less productive. You can blow a lifelong reputation for kindliness and civility with just one angry explosion; everyone will remember the outburst—and forget your years of patience!

So go ahead and write that angry letter to the colleague or administrator who did you wrong, if you feel you must. But don't send it. Procrastinate. Slip it into your desk drawer and take it out a few days later. In 99% of cases, you'll have cooled down, or settled the misunderstanding, and you can toss the letter, no harm done. If you're still upset, you can always send it. But *primo non nocere.*

If you've already said something that has hurt someone's feelings, or embarrassed them publicly, or you've fought with someone, do not procrastinate: Send a note of apology *right now.* Yes, right now; put this book down and send it. You'll be making two people feel better.

### *Primo Commendare*—First, Commend Someone

The best possible act you can do first thing when you sit down at your desk is **send someone a commendation**.

Remember the consultant who went out of her way to research a puzzling question for you, the nurse who caught what might have been a serious error, the administrator who went out on a limb to get your patient the needed resources? They'd love to receive a few words of appreciation. And don't forget to send copies to the chief of staff, chief of nursing services, and the other big honchos.

### The Commendation Letter

Recently a patient's family sent a letter thanking and commending a few of our nursing staff. Someone posted it on the office bulletin board. Reading it, I noticed that one of our newer nurses—who seemed to be having a tough time adjusting to the faster pace on that ward—was mentioned by name in the letter, and singled out for special praise. I told her about the letter (no one else had said anything to her), and led her over to the bulletin board.

As she read the letter, she started to glow with pride, and smiled a lovely smile of private joy and confidence that I had never seen on her face before. She stood up straighter, turned around, and to no one in particular said, sweetly and quietly, "Wow."

Since then, she's been doing great.

We're generally so stingy about sending commendations to each other, you'd think it might break our arm to write something nice about someone. Don't procrastinate about praise: Start now sending commendations regularly to people who deserve them, and the good effects will ripple out into your medical community. Morale will go up, other people will start sending commendations (you'll probably get one, too), the credentials files will get something good in them, quality will go up—and, believe me, the people who have received your written commendation will bend over backwards to serve you and your patients with special attention in the future. No one ever forgets praise.

It's a win-win-win that costs absolutely nothing—and by the way, neither does a smile in the morning to all you meet, and that works wonders, too. Don't feel like smiling? Do it anyway.

> A professional is someone who does their best
> when feeling their worst.

**Notes**

1. C. Lock, "What Value Do Computers Provide to NHS Hospitals?" *British Medical Journal* 312 (1996): 1,407–1,410.
2. "Giving a Clinic on Automating Records," *Health Data Management,* July 1996, 28–29.
3. F. Bazzoli, "Clinics Face a Daunting Task," *Health Data Management,* October 1996, 39–41.
4. J. Frieden, "Feds Targeting Managed Care Fraud," *Clinical Psychiatry News,* November 1997, 32.
5. "Productive Calling," *Success Magazine,* September 1994, 33.
6. T. Zwillich, "Know Algorithms to Get Treatments Authorized," *Clinical Psychiatry News,* June 1997, 34.
7. D. Green, "Reduce the Stress of Calling the Physician," *American Journal of Nursing,* September 1997, 49–51.
8. P.G. Churgin, "Compensating Physicians for Telephone Calls," letter, *Journal of the American Medical Association* 274, no. 3 (1995): 216.
9. S.Q. Wheeler and B. Siebelt, "How to Perform Telephone Triage," *Nursing 97,* July 1997, 37.
10. J. Manzo, *Surviving without a Secretary* (Menlo Park, CA: Crisp Publishers, 1996), 57.

## ✦ 6 ✦

# How to Rearrange Your Clinical Work for Higher Efficiency

You've set a personal goal, debrided your calendar, and eliminated or reduced some of the major time wasters.

Now you can concentrate on rearranging your remaining work in time and space so that you can do it faster and more efficiently.

The key here is to analyze your usual work patterns and then change them around to better fit your own optimum way of getting things done. This is a customizing job, so these suggestions will necessarily be more general than the others; you'll want to adapt them for your individual work style.

## Blocking

Blocking is something we do intuitively, to take advantage of the mind's basic tendency to get in a groove and stay there—the "cheaper-by-the-dozen" principle. It's usually more efficient to **stack up a block of similar things to be done at one sitting**, like saving your household bills for two weeks and then writing all the checks in one evening.

Blocking lets you stay in the rhythm of repetitive work and build momentum. We can switch to autopilot if the chores are similar and undemanding. Some surgeons have told me that rather than getting fatigued from doing more than one similar procedure in a day, they find that they actually get better and faster as they do several in a block.

If your paperwork dribbles in all day, and if none of it is emergent, you'll probably have your staff line it all up so you can go right through it. Ditto for phone calls. Some physicians block their paperwork into the last 30 minutes of the workday; others prefer to spread the unpleasant work more thinly through the day. Some physicians and surgeons block all their office visits into two or three weekdays, meetings into one afternoon, etc.

The exception: If you're already stressed, blocking your work may be a bad idea; variety and frequent changes from one type of work to another may serve you better. Experiment and decide for yourself.

If you've taken control of your schedule, you can more easily arrange for similar work to be clumped for your personal convenience and efficiency. This is such an easy thing to do that I'm surprised some docs don't seem to have thought of insisting that their staff block all their calls, or signatures, or orders, or certain types of patient exams. Insist that they have similar work all lined up before they call you.

## Chipping

Chipping is the reverse of blocking: You **chip off a little piece of a bigger block of work and do it in stages**. This works well for a big, onerous job that you'd otherwise put off indefinitely, or until you have to do it under the pressure of a deadline.

You already used chipping when you wrote down your personal professional goal, and then broke it down into smaller, doable steps or objectives—chips. By keeping after your goal daily, one chip at a time, you can change your entire professional life— achieve a whole new level of clinical expertise, e.g.

There was a man named Bunyan who said, "I can't write a book." A friend asked him, "Well, could you just write one page?" "Sure, I can write a page. Anyone can write a page." So John Bunyan wrote just one page a day, and finally he did create a book—*Pilgrim's Progress*—which became not only a best seller, but a classic, translated into over 40 languages. He wrote it in little chips, one page at a time.

### Traffic

The busy strip highway in our valley fills with traffic at certain hours of the day, and long lines of cars used to pile up at one or two large intersections. A few months ago they installed a half-dozen traffic lights at 200-yard intervals, and we cursed the new obstacles.

But the new traffic lights seem to have eliminated the congestion, and now the heavy traffic, broken up into chips, flows smoothly and unhindered.

I'm not sure of the principle involved, but breaking up long, unrelieved blocks of work into smaller chips can sometimes help your daily tasks go more smoothly and with less stress.

**Exercise 6–1** Analyze your work over a week, see which small tasks you or your staff can more conveniently block together in time, and try it. If your staff continue to feed you work in dribbles and spurts, explain to them that you can be more productive if they'll block together questions, orders, phone calls, paperwork, similar procedures, etc.

Find a bigger project you have not been able to start, and try breaking it down into smaller chips that you can do. Do the first chip, and then continue, one small chip at a time, until you're done.

## Pumped and Slumped

We know as physicians that everything inside our body has its own rhythm: our heart, our brain, our catecholamine secretion, etc. It shouldn't come as a surprise that our work has rhythms, also. And just as our own heart beats a little differently from everyone else's, our individual work rhythms are different, too.

My wife, for instance, will often start her most creative work around 11 at night, when I can barely muster the energy to drag myself off to bed. At 2 AM she'll still be working away on some project. But when I come bounding up at 7 AM, full of vim and vigor, she raises one sleepy eyelid just long enough to tell me to buzz off until a more decent hour.

Obviously, our daily work rhythms are different!

Osler recognized that some medical students were day people, and others were night people ("larks" and "owls"). He theorized that the larks ran higher temperatures early in the morning, and owls warmed up at night.[1]

These cycles also extend through the year. My wife becomes most productive in the winter months when it's cold, foggy, and rainy. At the first chilly blast, I'm off to Palm Springs to hibernate. Every summer just before my birthday I get a big energy surge, while she goes into a slump until the cool weather returns before her birthday in the winter.

Personally, I don't do my best work on Mondays. But by Tuesday I'm warmed up, and by Friday evening, when the staff parking lot is deserted, I'm at my most productive; I get a lot of my best work done late on Fridays.

If you **analyze your own work week for rhythms**, you'll spot some times when you're "pumped" and some times when you tend to be "slumped."

## Optimize Your Schedule

Once you know your slumped/pumped cycle, you can rearrange your schedule to squeeze out higher productivity. For instance, I often shunt busywork or boring meetings to Mondays, because that's a low-productivity time for me anyway. But if it's something involving creative thinking, I'll save it for Friday afternoon. If you find some of your work boring or difficult, try switching it to another time or a different day.

Also, optimize your schedule according to your individual work psychology. A busy friend in Chicago tells me he's so rushed during the week he can't get all his paperwork done. By Friday night he usually ends up with a big stack of charts left to work on. But he'll get them done then, no matter what, even if he has to stay late—because he doesn't want to meet those charts again on Monday morning, and ruin his week.

I tend to do just the opposite. Because my work rhythms tend to peak on Fridays, I purposely leave half-finished work on my desk Friday night, so that on Monday morning—when I slump—it will be easier for me to pick up where I left off. Other people like to do their hardest job first thing in the morning, so the rest of the day they can coast.

The point is: Be flexible, and **work with your natural rhythms**. Some physicians like to work after 6 PM when everyone else is gone, telephones and beepers are quiet, and they can get through a lot of solitary work quickly. Others find being alone in a darkened hospital or office a bit creepy, or they don't like the feeling of being at work while everyone else is home with their families. Some surgeons like to do their first case at 7 AM, others prefer a 10 AM start. Experiment with changing around your start times.

There's nothing sacred about two four-hour shifts. Some practitioners reportedly find they can get the same amount done in one uninterrupted shift of six or seven hours, junking the usual four-hour-plus-lunch-then-four-more-hours schedule. By eliminating pre-lunch and post-lunch slowdowns, they can save three hours a day—"six straight can equal eight."

On the other hand, stopping work for lunch may be vital to your sanity. At one large university medical center, residents are more or less ordered to get out of the building during lunch and stroll, play racquetball, or whatever. Having a midday break at that place is considered a must for residents' health.

Bottom line: Try flexing your own work time, to find what feels best.

 **Exercise 6–2** Observe your work patterns over a day (week, month), looking for cycles and rhythms. Then try shifting your schedule and calendar to fit these rhythms better.

Notice the rhythms of your team, your office staff, your partners, your patients. See if there are ways you can better mesh your work with their rhythms—or get them to mesh with yours.

Attitude change: Think flexible. Why should an unexpected 6:30 PM admission be such an annoyance? If we analyze why we get upset and feel stressed in such a situation, sometimes it turns out that we had been counting on getting finished with our work at a certain definite time—but that it actually won't mean the end of the world if we get home half an hour later than usual. The next time you find yourself rushing and cursing over an unexpected chore, try to remind yourself that you made your schedule, and you can simply choose to unmake it. The stress will disappear instantly (but you'll still have to do the chore).

## Focus, Focus

A few years back, my wife fell very ill with what turned out be a nasty atypical pneumonia. She seemed to be sinking, and I thought she was close to respiratory failure when I rushed her to our local hospital ER.

Luckily, the physician on duty was someone I personally knew to be an excellent clinician. A seasoned man, he was thorough and very focused. He got preliminary studies quickly, and by mid-afternoon had called a pulmonologist to come and take over my wife's case.

Then the shift changed.

The ER doctor who came on duty was nattily dressed, and he motored up in a sleek sports model. He sauntered around the room, bantered casually with some of the nurses, glanced at the charts, and then settled into a long conversation with a technician about baseball.

This second physician, it was clear to me, just wasn't focused on his patients. What worried me more, he wasn't focused on my wife—who was gravely ill and, as far as I knew, in mortal danger.

The first physician must have picked up on my anxiety, because instead of leaving at the end of his shift, he stayed with my wife until the pulmonologist arrived. Everything turned out OK, and after a few days in the hospital, my wife recovered.

But see how crucial it is—from our patients' point of view—that we **pay full attention**. We even use the phrase, "This person needs medical *attention*." So our patients expect it, and so do our co-workers.

There are also benefits for us if we're fully focused:

✦ We can get more work done in a given time, and our work will be of better quality, with fewer errors.

✦ We'll have less mental stress, and we'll be more optimistic, because our outside life is forgotten whenever we focus fully on our patients and their needs. (We can't do anything about our personal problems at that moment, anyway, except worry.) The poet–pediatrician William Carlos Williams wrote that he lost himself and became so absorbed in his patients' lives that "...nothing of myself affected me."[2(p.92)]

✦ When we fully concentrate, we're automatically "in flow," a sort of peak mental/emotional experience, which is closer to play than to work; so by staying fully concentrated we can literally turn our work into play.

✦ Some physicians claim they've developed an ability to focus intently on a clinical problem until they "see" the solution. There is certainly no question that the best medical students, the best residents, and the best practitioners have in common the habit of very good concentration.

✦ When you're fully focused and concentrated, other people around you can work with more focused attention also; it's sort of infectious, as is being scattered.

✦ The highly focused and concentrated physician is more powerful, commanding, and effective in all her interpersonal interactions; it's the difference between a flashlight and a laser. When you give your orders and requests with fully focused attention, people respond more carefully and more accurately. So being fully focused cuts down on re-work and misunderstandings.

### One Thing at a Time

Although trying to do two things at once may sound like a good way to save time, avoid it. Most of us can actually keep more balls in the air if we **focus fully on one thing at a time**. While we can do a small amount of parallel mental processing, we're actually more efficient at single-channel tasks. Trying to focus on two things at once means we're neglecting one of them.

Some psychologists recommend "compartmentalizing"—keeping our private and professional lives separated by a mental firewall so they don't interfere with each other. This is particularly important if we're raising children, or just trying to have a satisfying family life.

The best course, suggested by the teacher Kirpal Singh: **At work, be fully at work; at home, be fully at home.** Our patients and our families both deserve our full attention.

There's the story of an engineer who built big towers for a living. At one point in his career he began to hang out with his crew after quitting time, instead of going home. They sat and gabbed, and the long evenings passed pleasantly but unproductively. His mentor confronted him one day with the question, "Tell me—how tall are the towers you build in the evenings?"

Which is not to say that we can't spend break time (or time waiting for an OR) relaxing with colleagues, or socializing with our staff. Such moments can actually be very enriching; they build our relationships, and relax and recharge us. Since some manual procedures can be done on automatic, light chat during undemanding work is common. But in general, most physicians feel that we're in this profession to help our patients, not for a social life, so we need to keep our eye focused on the ball—not on baseball.

 **Exercise 6–3** Measure how long you are able to keep your mind on a given task before you become distracted, start thinking about something else, and lose your concentration. Time yourself using a watch with a second hand. Try the exercise in a noisy clinical workspace. Try it also in a quiet, private place. You can use counting by threes as a task. Don't be surprised if you find your concentration span is short.

To improve your concentration, consider taking up a pursuit that demands total concentration, such as yoga, chess, tai chi, a martial art, or—perhaps the best of all—meditation. Do it every day, and re-measure your concentration span after a few weeks.

> Try doing only one clinical task at a time, concentrat-
> ing on it fully. See if you can actually get more done,
> with fewer slips, by being fully focused on only one
> task at a time.

All of us have good attention—if we didn't, we never could
have made it through our medical training. We learned how to
force ourselves to focus on a lecture after being up all night on the
wards, and later we used the same skill to keep our attention focused on our work during long surgical procedures or late-night
medical watches.

Whatever we can do to strengthen our attention will help us be
more accurate and effective in everything we do. Contrary to what
some psychologists say, the habit of focusing attention can be
transferred from one task to another. I doubt I could have practiced my specialty—which involves daily contact with very disturbed individuals—without meditating every morning for the
past 25 years.

> "Success in any sphere is the result of sustained
> effort and concentrated attention."
>
> Rajinder Singh[3(p.6)]

Of course, **avoid mixing work with anything that destroys
or weakens your concentration**. Not only are drugs, alcohol,
and fatigue on this list, but also less obvious stuff like moods (anxiety, depression, anger), illness, hunger, pain, etc. Pregnancy, recent research shows, can be associated with some mild decre-
ment in attention (probably in new fathers, too!).

Finally: If we can succeed at keeping our attention focused
steadily on a given goal, project, or clinical field for years, then we
can achieve something great.

Newton and Napoleon

All the great achievers of history have had unusually good attention. It's said of Sir Isaac Newton that he was sitting under a tree studying math when a brass band went by. Someone asked him, "Which way did the band go?" and Newton answered, "What band?" His attention was that good.

Similarly, Napoleon was so focused that on the morning of a huge battle when his generals, fretting and worried, came to discuss tactics, he was coolly working on some papers. "Oh, that battle," the emperor reportedly said. "That's at 9 o'clock; it's only 8 o'clock now."

## Commuting

A surgeon spoke up at a recent seminar to complain about his stressful daily commute. Then an internist across the room said that personally he enjoyed his commute, and considered it the most stress-free time of his working day. I asked the two docs how long their commutes were. "A half hour," answered the stressed-out surgeon. "About two and one-half hours, on a good day," said the happy internist.

A case of different lives, different drives.

If you must commute, it makes sense to get the most comfortable and reliable car you can afford; get rid of that junker left over from your residency. Find a more scenic route, if you can. A neurosurgeon told me he considered his one-hour commute along a beautiful lakeside his daily unpaid vacation. Research does suggest that many people tend to feel good while they're driving (perhaps because they're in control of an efficient piece of machinery).

Six months ago, a friend cut out the 60-mile commute he was making to a neighboring county. He tells me he now has much more time with his growing children, while added office visits in his home county have already made up for the lost work. Now he plans also to drop the 25-mile commute he's making into the city, and confine his practice entirely to one office and two nearby hospitals.

Although you may not find your commute noxious, take a moment to consider whether it's the most productive way you can be spending your time—and whether it's possible to **simplify your life by working closer to home**.

### Hey! What About Our Patients' Time?

Business analysts tell us that our profession is not only less efficient, but also less consumer driven than other more modern industries. The trick, we are told, is to be both at the same time. That's a pretty good trick.

Which brings us to the patient waiting in our office for a visit or a procedure. Customer satisfaction surveys indicate that short waiting times are important to our patients, yet overscheduling is routine in busy offices where work flow has to be maintained. Most of our patients (including women) now have demanding work schedules, so the opportunity cost of waiting to see us can be very high.

What these surveys don't say is that most patients are dissatisfied with curt and casual visits, no matter how quickly they're seen, and most patients will wait longer to see a practitioner whose clinical—and interpersonal—skills are higher than average. On the other hand, if your patient waits 90 minutes and then perceives you as preoccupied or uncaring, you may not see her again.

Scattered throughout this book, but especially in Part 4, you'll discover practical techniques for increasing your patients' satisfaction under speed-up. Also, as your own efficiency improves (with less time lost in interruptions, phone calls, paperwork, rework, etc.), waiting times will go down. Your office staff can also come up with innovative and more efficient arrangements, and we'll discuss teamwork at length in Part 4.

## Take Charge of Your Workspace

Even if we don't commute long distances, most physicians these days do have to move around a lot. In any given day we may be in our private office, several examining rooms and hospital rooms, a few nursing stations, a meeting room, our car, the OR, perhaps the ER or the ICU, etc. It's only common sense that each of these workspaces should be arranged to maximize the efficient use of our time there—but this is not always true.

Take some time to **make sure that all the places where you work regularly have been arranged specifically for your convenience and efficiency.** Something as obvious as being sure the instruments or forms that you tend to use most frequently are kept where you can get your hands on them quickly will speed your work and cut down on frustration. If you haven't already, **do a walk-through of your workspace with staff to rearrange it for speed and efficiency.**

Sometimes when I first come into a clinical workspace I'm amazed to find that vacation leave requests or legal forms or someone's magazine have been placed in the front of files where clinical materials ought to be. I set things right immediately.

The same goes for our charts—if the charts at your hospital or clinic are not handy for you to use, call the medical records committee and get them changed. You're the major creator and user of the chart, and it should be arranged for your convenience. Simpler is better, and usually you can have a lot of the non-clinical stuff filed elsewhere. If you use those charts for years, the seconds saved if you **have all charts well organized for your work style** will add up.

If you're already using some form of electronic clinical data system, don't assume that it's set up for your maximum efficiency. In working with computer software people, I've been struck by how little they generally know about the work we do, and how we usually do it. If you can see ways to improve the system so it works better for you, let your data systems people know. If you run into resistance to your requests, remind everyone how often you need patient information in emergencies, so everything must be laid out for quick access by you.

## Your Office, Your Mess

Your private office is an unsightly mess? You're not the Lone Ranger. It's not necessarily neatness that counts: Professional office arrangers say that if you can lay your hands on whatever you're looking for in a short period of time, then it doesn't matter what your private office looks like.

Many practitioners use the so-called "hemorrhoid" system of filing: everything in piles. Our youngest daughter keeps all her stuff in piles—on the floor. She makes a pile of books to the left, then one to the right, walks between them, and can say, "Now I've been through all these books." When we ask her to clean up the mess, she insists she knows where everything is, and disturbing the mess would ruin her system. Since she's getting higher grades than I ever did, I can't criticize her arrangement.

My daughter's stacks of stuff illustrate a general principle of organizing space, which we've already discussed under organizing your schedule: As messy or chaotic as a space may seem to someone else, if you have organized it that way, and you're the person who works there, chances are it's organized efficiently—for *your* work patterns. Nothing is more frustrating than coming into your office one morning to discover that some neatnik has gone through and relocated and relabeled everything so you can't find what you need. They usually think they're doing you a favor. They're not. Discourage such people strongly, and make them put everything back.

On the other hand, if you ever do feel the need to have someone else make your office space better organized, there are professional office organizers you can hire. They have their own national association, and several office managers have told me they are worth their fee in increased efficiency for your whole team.

As part of the research for the productivity seminar, I called and consulted with one of these professional office organizers, let's call her Naomi Neatly (almost her real name). Ms. Neatly was very strict with me on the phone; her tone reminded me of my third-grade teacher. She made it clear that if she did reorganize my office for me, I would have to follow her instructions, and observe discipline. I began to have the distinct feeling that if I didn't do exactly what she told me to, she might spank me, so I dropped the whole project.

But if you go in for that sort of thing, you'll find these pros in the Yellow Pages under "Organizing Services and Systems."

## The High-Efficiency OR

If you do much work in an OR, you've noticed that these workspaces are getting more and more crowded by machines, leaving less and less room for humans to work in. Fortunately, a new discipline of operating-room ergonomics is starting up, researching the best heights and distances for tables and video monitors, the most efficient angles for standing and bending, etc.[4] Considering how many surgeons are reporting problems with stress injuries, this is a valuable new development. If you can't access the research, you could certainly **make a careful appraisal of your surgical workspace yourself** to see if it can be improved ergonomically for your comfort and efficiency. Check into having more efficient and productive instruments for the procedures you do most frequently. One recent study showed that a well-designed laparoscopic device increased surgeons' efficiency by 20%.[5]

### A Pearl

It was, as I recall, our very first day out of the labs and lecture halls, when we crossed over to the hospital to begin our clinical clerkships. Our team started out on pathology rotation, and we showed up at the morgue after lunch in our brand new, bright white coats, eager to learn.

"Alright, I'm going to start by giving you a pearl, and I never want you to forget it," began the crusty senior resident as we flocked worshipfully around the autopsy table.

"This pearl is something you won't find in any textbook, and you won't hear it in any lecture—but I guarantee it will save you trouble every day for the rest of your life in medicine."

We whipped out our pocket notebooks and clicked our pens excitedly, waiting to receive…our first clinical pearl! Would it be the arcane key to making lightning-swift diagnoses? Some rule of thumb for calculating unerringly accurate drug doses? We waited, and he spoke.

"Here's the pearl: Never do any procedure standing up that you can do sitting down."

Not too profound. In fact a bit homely. Yet I've never quite forgotten the advice, I do use it every day—and it has indeed saved me a lot of trouble over the past 35 years.

**Exercise 6–4** Circle the suggestions below (taken from the preceding chapters) which you will try out in your own practice. Add your own suggestions at the end of this list in the spaces provided. Keep this book in your office and refer back to this list when you have a moment. Analyze which suggestions are working best for you, and consider whether some others on the list may be worth trying.

Perhaps only a few of these suggestions will fit your particular practice style. Try to implement the ones that make the most sense to you, however, and you'll discover that other ways to cut down on wasted time (and replace it with more productive time) will start suggesting themselves to you. After a while, you'll become an expert on using your time efficiently.

1. Choose a personal professional goal.

2. Write down your goal on a card.

3. Carry the card with you and check it every working day.

4. Work on your goal first thing every day.

5. Put in time on your goal daily.

6. Prioritize those activities that relate to your goal.

7. Take charge of your own schedule.

8. Say no to all unreasonable intrusions on your schedule.

9. Systematically take items off your schedule.

10. Don't start any project you won't definitely finish.

11. Finish one thing every day.

12. Don't allow any unreasonable interruptions while you're working.

13. Buy a huge wastebasket for your office, and use it.

14. Stick to some methodical technique of paper-work reduction.

15. Don't go to any meeting unless it's confirmed.

16. Eliminate habit and ritual meetings.

17. Get on the minutes-only list.

18. Have someone go to meetings in your place.

19. Be careful about how you use the phone.

20. In general, avoid the delusion of procrastination.

21. Procrastinate on chores that you'll have to re-do later.

22. Procrastinate to avoid shady actions.

23. Procrastinate when about to act in anger.

24. Send commendations to co-workers.

25. Block similar tasks and do them all at one sitting.

26. Bite off little pieces of a big job, and do it in stages.

27. Analyze your work week for "pumped and slumped" times.

28. Work flexibly, with your natural rhythms.

29. Pay full attention to your work.

30. Focus on one thing at a time.

31. At work, be fully at work; at home, be fully at home.

32. Avoid anything that weakens your attention.

33. Simplify your life by working close to home.

34. Make sure all your workspaces have been arranged for your convenience and efficiency.

35. Do a walk-through with staff.

36. Have all charts well organized for your work style.

37. Make an ergonomic appraisal of your surgical workplace.

(add your own suggestions here)

_____

_____

_____

_____

**Notes**

1. W. Osler, *Aequanimitas* (Philadelphia, PA: Blakiston, 1932), 408.

2. R. Jorgenson and F. Shroser, *A College Treasury: Prose* (New York: Charles Scribner & Sons, 1967), 92.

3. R. Singh, *Inner and Outer Peace Through Meditation* (Rockport, MA: Element Books, Inc., 1996), 6.

4. R. Berguer and Z. Szabo, "Ergonomics: The Link Between the Surgical Team and the Operating Room Environment," in *Proceedings, U.C. Davis 3rd Annual Surgical Update* (1997), 127–135.

5. D. Wallwiener et al., "Multifunctional Instrument for Operative Laparoscopy," *Endoscopic Surgery and Allied Technologies* 3 (1995): 119–124.

# Part 3

# Knowledge Management for Physicians

"Everyone is ignorant, only on different subjects."

Will Rogers

# ✦ 7 ✦

# Take Control
# of Your Clinical
# Knowledge Base

You're now saving anywhere from a few minutes to a few hours every week by assertively managing your use of time. Up to this point, it necessarily has been slash-and-burn; by force of will you've cut away the unproductive undergrowth that was choking your schedule.

Now you have some breathing space in which to think about what you're doing. The thesis of this book is that we can become much more productive by investing some of our time and effort into analyzing our daily practice habits and making them less wasteful, then reinvesting the additional time and effort saved to become still more productive, etc.—thereby setting in motion an upward spiral of ever-increasing personal efficiency and effectiveness. If this sounds like an attractive plan for increasing your productivity even more, let's move on and learn to better manage our second tool: Knowledge.

## More (Useful) Knowledge Makes Your Work More Efficient

Because we're under pressure to speed up, we have less opportunity these days to get the knowledge we need to do our clinical work most efficiently. Yet, if you have just the right bit of clinical skill or knowledge available at just the right moment, you can work more quickly, and with better outcomes. Think about how fast, sure, and effective your routine clinical work is—but how you have to slow down when you're working in a less familiar area, where your knowledge base and skills are sketchy.

Since individual medical practice essentially consists of knowledge applied over time, or $K \times T$, you can see that—within limits—the more usable knowledge you have available (higher $K$), the less time and effort (lower $T$) you'll have to spend accomplishing a given quantity and quality of clinical work.

> ❝Send a patient to a doctor who knows what he or she is doing, and it will cost you half of what it would otherwise.❞
>
> Benjamin Safirstein, MD[1](p.12)

So although you spend only 5% of your working time getting and maintaining your clinical knowledge, what you do during those few hours a month will have a huge effect on how productive you are during the other 95%. Having the best and most usable knowledge in the right place at the right time is like using a bulldozer instead of a pick and shovel.

## Too Much Knowledge

Physicians complain they have too little time, but the complaint is just the opposite with knowledge: These days, there's just *too much* knowledge out there for any one person to master. Because as much new medical knowledge is created every month as was previously created in decades, we have to learn (and unlearn) more in our lifetimes than any other generation of physicians ever dreamed of.

But too much available knowledge is just another way of saying we have too little time in which to sift out the practical core of knowledge we really need, and absorb it. So the general principles of effective knowledge management are similar to those we've already learned to use in managing our time:

1. **Take personal control of your own continuing professional education.** Just as you first had to take back control of your schedule and calendar to manage your time, start taking active, personal control of your most valuable professional assets: your knowledge and skills.

2. **Customize your own professional education to meet your actual needs.** No one except you can efficiently manage your personal knowledge base, because your individual pattern of skills, learning preferences, clinical style, and patient mix is unique to you. The trick is to know exactly what your actual needs are.

3. **Cut out wasteful learning habits**, especially random acquisition of clinical knowledge that may or may not be of value in your practice. Your personal knowledge base is much too important to entrust to serendipity.

4. **Become maximally efficient at acquiring**, maintaining, and using clinical **knowledge**. Sorry, but the old ways won't cut it any more, as comfortable and familiar as they are. The world of knowledge has changed radically in the past few years, and we have to change, too. For openers, we have to change the setting of our personal knowledge software—our brain—from "browse" to "search."

## *Scientia Potentia*

Knowledge is power.

Your power to help, to heal, to influence—all your power as a physician grows directly out of your specialized knowledge.

Isn't saying you're a physician just another way of saying that you've acquired certain types of knowledge that most other people don't have? Medicine is almost a perfect meritocracy, based solely on knowledge and skill: Whether you're a man or a woman; black, white, brown, or yellow; a Hindu or a Christian or a Jew; come from a rich or poor family, or from Meerut or Miami—none of it makes any difference to the patient waiting for you to do a procedure on him. He couldn't care less whether you're a Buddhist, a Republican, or a vegetarian; his only question is, Do you have enough knowledge and skill to do this procedure successfully?

It's illegal for any person to practice medicine without proof that he has acquired specialized knowledge (credentials). This monopoly is in the interest of society, since it guarantees that only the brightest and best-trained people will treat patients. Ethics, altruism, ambition, and stamina are all desiderata of the medical life—but no one becomes a physician without being able to master the enormous constellation of knowledge and skills required of every doctor.

### Weeded Out

In the first few months of medical school, I shared a cadaver in Gross Anatomy with three hard-driving, ambitious young people. On a late-autumn afternoon, one of our foursome came by the anatomy lab to announce sadly that he had been asked to leave school; he just wasn't up to it intellectually. We never saw him again.

## We'll Need Even More (Useful) Knowledge in the Future

You may recall the opening scene of the classic French comedy film, *Mr. Hulot's Holiday*: A vacation-bound crowd is waiting on a railway station platform when the garbled voice over the loud-speaker seems to announce a track change. The whole crowd scurries down some stairs and through a tunnel to reappear on another platform. Then the garbled loudspeaker voice drones again, and they all rush back through the tunnel to the original platform. The voice again, and again they all hurry back to the second platform.

At last the train steams slowly in—on a different track altogether.

We seem to be going through somewhat the same scenario in health care. After decades of increasing specialization, MCOs switched to generalist-gatekeeper models. Now we're rushing back in the other direction: Seers are predicting that the future of our profession lies in the direction of more, not less, specialization. Chronic diseases like diabetes are astronomically expensive to treat (hundreds of billions of dollars each year), so in a few years, most diabetics may be managed by specialist teams in "boutique" clinics that deal exclusively and in depth with all aspects of the disease. Patients who need a procedure will be referred to centers of excellence whose physicians do nothing but that one procedure—at which they are super-experts. Specialized "hospitalists" will take over when your patient needs to be hospitalized, and so on.

If this disease-management/center-of-excellence approach really is the wave of the future, then to make it work, physicians will need to acquire and maintain highly specialized knowledge in depth. We'll need more efficient systems of personal knowledge management. (We'll also need the ability to work better in teams—which we'll get to in Part 4.) But no matter what your practice is like, useful knowledge has such a short half-life these days that methodically updating your skills and learning new techniques is the only way to guarantee yourself a secure future in our profession.

Since managing our knowledge is so crucial, it's surprising that we're not very efficient at doing it. Much of our so-called continuing education after we leave training isn't continuous at all; it's quite discontinuous, a series of random, hit-or-miss efforts to somehow keep up with new knowledge.

Part of our problem may be that we don't have a good grasp of what our current personal knowledge base looks like. Also, we may think that CME is like medical school. Finally, we may be going about our acquisition of new knowledge backward, and using outdated or unsuitable methods.

## The First Surprise: Your Personal Knowledge Base Is Shrinking Faster Than You Think

When you started pre-med, the knowledge you acquired first was general, and not particularly new: the basic anatomy of vertebrates (remember that dogfish?), the fundamentals of physics, chemistry, and so forth. You went on in medical school to sample the whole corpus of clinical medicine and surgery, spending some time on every service, and demonstrating some minimal skill in everything from rectal exams to the diagnosis of schizophrenia.

The area of the rectangle in Figure 7–1 represents all the available medical knowledge in the world. Ideally, a physician is expected to know everything there is to know about the human body. That's not possible—but it means ignorance can never be an excuse.

What you did get, as represented by the dark area in Figure 7–1, was a little thin, but it was as wide as possible, so when you graduated you knew as much as you ever would about the broad spectrum of medicine and surgery.

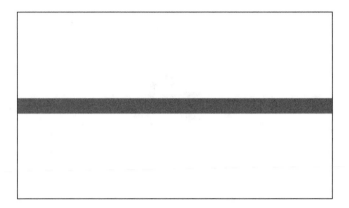

**Figure 7–1** Your personal knowledge base in medical school.

But maybe right from the first you knew you were going into plastic surgery; between bouts of studying anatomy you probably devoured the plastic surgery journals, admiring all those skin folds and tubes. Whatever your eventual choice of residency—family practice, internal medicine, pediatrics, psychiatry—you started at some point accumulating extra knowledge in that area. So your personal knowledge base had a little hump in it, even before you finished med school (Figure 7–2).

Then as a resident you immersed yourself in mastering every aspect of your specialized corner of medicine or surgery, until your knowledge base had grown a big hump like the one in Figure 7–3.

That was only the beginning of your learning. Since getting out into practice, you've spent years honing your expertise by handling 4,000 patient visits a year (on average), by reading and thinking and discussing, by taking more specialized courses, etc. Your hump has now grown into a lofty spire that reaches almost to the edge of the envelope of existing knowledge in your field (Figure 7–4).

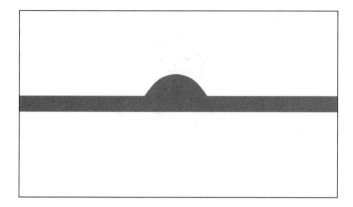

**Figure 7–2** Your personal knowledge base in medical school, with field of special interest.

---

If you're working daily in your field, you've probably gotten to that point where sometimes it's not just a question of whether *you* know a given fact or technique, but a question of whether *anyone* knows it; you're now working often at the cutting edge of knowl-

---

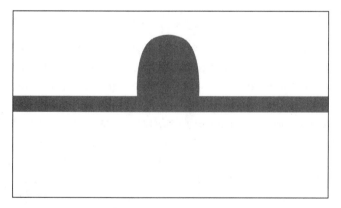

**Figure 7–3** Your personal knowledge base after completing residency/fellowship.

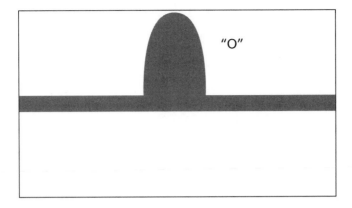

**Figure 7–4** Your personal knowledge base after 5–15 years in practice. "O" represents highly specialized knowledge that does not connect to your knowledge base.

edge in your chosen area. This happens to many of us in the natural course of our careers. If we keep up our training, take on more complex and difficult cases, and pay attention, our practical knowledge grows apace.

Meanwhile, we all keep up with general medicine and surgery outside our own field as best we can—but since our practice is limited, we'll inevitably lose some of the breadth we had in med school. So now we have a fairly broad knowledge base and a lovely, lofty spire of highly specialized knowledge in our field. That's now.

## The Knowledge Implosion (Why CME Is Crucial)

But just look where we would end up—say, four years from now—if we just maintained that same knowledge base (Figure 7–5). It looks at first glance like our personal knowledge base has shrunk again to almost nothing. Actually, it hasn't changed at all. What has happened is that the universe of available medi-

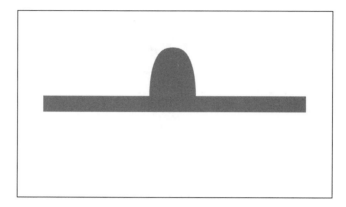

**Figure 7–5** Your personal knowledge base after four years without updating by regular CME.

cal knowledge has expanded exponentially during those four years, as new knowledge in every field of medicine goes on multiplying at the astounding rate of 100% every two years.[2] Our personal knowledge base has shrunk in comparison with what is now known.

We're all familiar with this constant pushing of the envelope of knowledge. Each of us knows that our own specialty has changed radically in the past few years because of some major new advance: In surgery, it's laparoscopic procedures; in psychiatry, all-new drugs for depression, dementia, mania, and schizophrenia; in infectious disease, protease inhibitors; and on and on.

There's so much new knowledge in medicine and surgery constantly displacing the old, that it's estimated half of what you learned in medical school is outdated after 10 years (some say eight), then half of what's left is outdated in another 10 years, and so on (Figure 7–6). If you've been out of school for about 20 years, less than one-fourth of what you learned then is still current. And of the fourth that's still useful, you've naturally forgotten a good

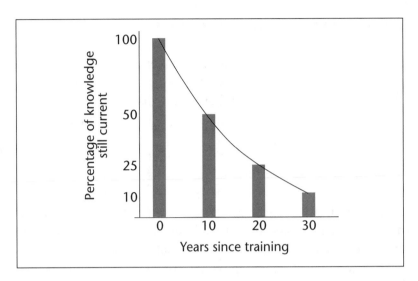

**Figure 7–6** Decay rate of medical knowledge.

portion. (If you don't think you've forgotten a lot and if you don't mind a nasty shock, pull down a copy of *Preparing for the MCAT* at your local bookstore, and try to answer even one of the sample questions.)

The good news is, a certain amount of what we learned in school was crap, anyway, so losing it isn't a big tragedy.

The bad news is *each of us risks becoming totally out of touch with the state of our art, unless we systematically pursue further clinical training all the years of our medical career.*

This point was driven home to me personally a few years ago while studying for my specialty boards. Psychoanalysis had been a heavy part of my residency curriculum, so naturally I searched for the section on psychoanalysis in the newest psychiatry text. To my shock, my entire four years of residency training in psycho-analysis had shrunk down to just seven pages in the new text-book—the remaining 900 pages, mostly on biological psychiatry, was pretty much all new since I finished residency.[3]

### Knowledge Travels Faster and Wider

Besides the rapid decay rate of our personal clinical knowledge, we have to deal with two brand new problems: electronic speedup of knowledge dissemination means new knowledge has a faster velocity than ever; it also means that new knowledge now spreads to a much wider audience.

Your peers and your patients know about any new clinical technique or discovery days, or even hours, after it's announced. And they expect you to know about it. Patients judge their physicians at least partially on how up-to-date our knowledge and techniques are. This makes sense; we all want to use the latest and best available skills in our practice, for our patients' sake.

So how can we become maximally efficient at getting the new knowledge and skills we need? As a first step, we need to analyze the CME process and see what it is—and what it isn't.

### The Second Surprise: Your CME Has Little to Do with TME (Traditional Medical Education)

Much formal CME is given at medical centers, and often by medical school faculty. But I'll go out on a limb here, and risk annoying my academic friends: Pedagogic-didactic medical school-type education and CME for the busy practitioner have little in common, except that they may happen in the same buildings. They are, or should be, very different processes. Think about these facts:

Medical schools, as part of the traditional university, were designed a century ago to give young college graduates a broad, standardized preparation for practicing medicine. These schools were not designed to help us busy practitioners maintain the individualized set of practical clinical skills that we need at this stage of our careers.

In medical school we were all fed pretty much the same basic curriculum, since we all started out with equal levels of ignorance, and since we all needed to end up with at least the same basic minimum of knowledge. But your brain is not infinitely expandable, so now you have to make sure the available room gets filled with knowledge that is of maximum value to you. You also don't have time to spend on getting knowledge that won't help you do your clinical work.

> **"In the blizzard of information swirling around us, it is easy to lose sight of our ultimate goal—finding ways to help our patients."**
>
> A.F. Shaughnessy, PharmD
> D.C. Slawson, MD[4(p.2,156)]

When you were in med school and residency you worked in a teaching hospital or clinic, where every day you had access to teaching rounds, lectures, professors, attendings, preceptors, senior house staff, clinical bull sessions, libraries full of journals, a medical bookstore, and similar resources.

Now you're out in the world, probably miles from the nearest medical center. Perhaps you're the sole practitioner in your specialty. Isolated from the teaching hospital's abundant learning opportunities, you're going to have to set up your own system of self-education.

In fact, you're the only one who can do this. Since no medical educator can possibly know (1) how much you learned in med school, residency, and beyond, and what you've forgotten; (2) what your unique practice is like; (3) where the holes are in your grasp of needed current knowledge and skills; and (4) whether you have knowledge in depth, no standardized academic curriculum can possibly fit all your needs. So to be maximally efficient, you have to commit yourself to take over the serious job of designing and executing your own lifelong CME program. This is something no one else can do for you.

Now let's look at how we can become more efficient consumers and users of clinical knowledge.

---

### Notes

1. B. Safirstein, Interview, *Physician Practice Options,* September 1997, 12–13.
2. M. Hotvedt, "Continuing Medical Education: Actually Learning Rather Than Simply Listening," letter, *Journal of the American Medical Association* 275 (1996): 1,637–1,638.
3. H. Kaplan et al., *Kaplan and Sadock's Synopsis of Psychiatry* (Baltimore, MD: Williams & Wilkins, 1994), 824–828.
4. A.F. Shaughnessy and D.C. Slawson, "Getting the Most from Review Articles," *American Family Physician* 55, no. 6 (1997): 2,155–2,160.

# ✦ 8 ✦

# How to Get Rid of Your Journal Pile

To start managing your unique knowledge base more efficiently, **methodically analyze all of your CME activities to make sure they are maximally useful in your actual practice**. What is of little or no use you can eliminate and replace in your personalized curriculum with more valuable activities. Then, **actively seek and use educational materials that fit your unique needs**—which may not necessarily be the needs of an expert to lecture you today about his research, or of a drug company to sell you their product.

For example, an internist told me that for 15 years she had been learning and relearning the treatment of a rare fungal disease. Because the treatment methods for this disease keep changing, CME providers almost always include them in the standard medical review course. So every year or two she dutifully spent many CME hours learning the latest techniques in some detail.

Until one day it hit her: In her practice, she never saw any cases of that disease. Most of her patients were not at risk for contracting it, and she wasn't keeping up the minimal volume to be adept at handling a case.

Now she no longer tries to be an expert in this illness that she never sees, and instead spends the freed-up CME hours getting more proficient in treating the diseases she does see every day. If she runs into a case, she'll refer it or get the needed knowledge JIT (just in time) from her knowledge network, depending on the difficulty of the case. She says she saves time, and her clinical knowledge base is stronger for what she actually does every day in her office.

> What we learn in a lecture room but never use in our practice evaporates quickly. The converse is also true: What we use, we won't lose.

In medical school, we were full-time students and had the luxury of spending almost all of our time in getting new knowledge. Obviously, we busy practitioners have much less time and opportunity in which to absorb new knowledge. However, the fact that we're now working every day at patient care does give us one big advantage in managing our continuing education: We can see much more clearly our need for knowledge, and which knowledge we need.

### Learning Backwards

A pediatrics professor once confessed: "We do this whole medical education thing backwards. We try to fill students' brains with pathology, differential diagnosis, electrolyte formulas, drug doses, and such, and hope they'll still remember some of it by the time they get out on the wards and see some patients.

"We should be doing it exactly the other way around: first, let a medical student sit by the bed of a dying child for a few days, desperately trying to figure out what to do to save that child's life. Then they'll be motivated to learn differential diagnosis, pathophysi-

ology, pharmacology, differential therapeutics—and
everything else they really need to know."

The place to learn a foreign language is not in a lecture hall
memorizing lists of verbs on a blackboard; that's the slow, painful
way. Instead, spend some time living in that country, actually
needing to use that language every moment of the day—and
you'll learn it quickly and effortlessly.

Similarly, there is a certain time and situation when each of us is
especially receptive to learning and using a given chunk of new
clinical knowledge. Because as practitioners we're more interested in taking care of patients than we are in intellectual acquisi-
tions, we're most motivated to learn when we're faced with an
actual case—when we need to know something, we're best prepared to learn it.

Adult-learning experts call this "the teachable moment."

A huge multiplying effect in learning speed and effectiveness
results when you **hook up your educational activities directly
to your actual caseload**.

Recently, for instance, two colleagues attended the same seminar on new drugs in their field. Afterward, one said he hadn't been
able to follow the speaker, and had learned little or nothing. The
other physician said she thought the speaker was superb, and she
had picked up some valuable new information.

It turned out that this second doc had put several patients on
the new drugs, had recently noticed some possible problems, and
needed the information badly. But to the first doc the seminar was
an abstraction: He as yet had no patients on the drugs, so he
wasn't ready for that knowledge at that moment.

In systems terms, we would do well to JIT portions of our knowledge supply, the way Japanese auto makers JIT their parts sup-
plies. The most efficient way for most of us to acquire usable
knowledge is close to the point in time and space we need it most.

Research confirms that we retain more if we learn in a situation similar to the situation in which we're going to use the knowledge.

Surgeons commonly JIT their knowledge. If there's a procedure on his schedule that he hasn't done for a while, a surgeon will usually haul out a book or a recent article and review the anatomy. He may rehearse the procedure in his mind, step by step, visualizing the variations and pitfalls, and how he'll respond. He'll do this just before he performs the surgery itself, knowing instinctively that this is the best time to get the needed knowledge into his head and his hands.

### Your Personal Clinical Coach

Having an unfamiliar surgical procedure on your schedule is a pretty clear signal that you need to brush up, but usually it's difficult to be aware of exactly what you don't know. To make your personal knowledge acquisition more efficient, first **have a clearer idea of what it is you actually need to learn**.

When high-level athletes or performers are trying to maximize their efficiency, they hire a private coach to watch carefully what they do, analyze their weaknesses, and show them how to improve. A few years ago, when I started giving seminars professionally, I found a coach who was able to tell me in a couple of hours exactly what I was doing wrong during my programs, and how to correct these deficiencies.

Wouldn't it be ideal if you could have a private, confidential clinical coach follow you around ten hours a day, observe minutely every bit of clinical work you do, and then arrange for any deficiencies in your skills and knowledge to be corrected? Sure it would...except that there is no such person as a clinical coach. Even if there were, he couldn't analyze your practice in sufficient depth, because he would need to read your mind (that's where your decision making goes on). Since a private coach can't do the job, you'll have to do it yourself: Analyze your daily practice, locate areas that need strengthening, and arrange for appropriate training. Luckily, it's simpler than it sounds.

 **Exercise 8–1  Keep a "needs" card in your pocket at all times** during your work day. (Use the back of your Goal card.) On it, briefly note down:

- Types of cases that have puzzled you (or in which you've made an error)

- Facts you needed to know but didn't (whether in your field of expertise, or not)

- Any questions that have come up in your mind about patients you actually see

- Any procedures that you found slow, difficult, or that *you put off doing.*

Get this card out when you go to your journal pile or to the medical library, and use it to guide your reading.

Also use it when you're picking lectures and courses to attend, and when you're ordering tapes or going online.

Take your Needs card (or send a summary of it) to your CME Committee, so your real clinical needs will help decide future educational programs at your association meeting, hospital, or clinic.

Also, share what's on your card with others in your knowledge network (see below), so they know what articles to clip for you. Discuss what's on your card with them, and pick their brains for knowledge and skills you need to upgrade—or find out from them who has the skills you need, and seek them out.

> If some one item (or related items) keeps coming up
> over and over on your Needs card, be prompt about
> getting retrained and checked out in that area; you've
> found a gap in your clinical knowledge base.

Different items on your Needs card will call for different educational remedies:

✦ If you just need to brush up on NIDDM, e.g., you'll go to a recent textbook (be aware of the one- to three-year time lag for getting new information into textbooks) or a review article in your file (but many review articles lag behind the most recent findings, also).

✦ If you need to answer a knotty question about a particular patient, you'll most likely call someone in your knowledge network or your mentor, or search MEDLINE.

✦ If it's a particular procedure you need to sharpen, you'll want to attend a hands-on workshop through your specialty association or a university, etc.

✦ If you're not just brushing up, but instead need to master a whole new area of knowledge, you'll want a course or a series of courses, plus maybe some multimedia aids, and the like.

Don't be surprised if your Needs card doesn't necessarily list things you're interested in. Reviewing the diagnosis of Ehlers-Danlos syndrome may not be your idea of fun—but if your card shows this is a subject you need to brush up on because you are running into it, **do what your card says**. Research suggests that physicians actually learn better when we're given assignments, rather than randomly pursuing our own interests.[1] So it's up to us mature practitioners to assign educational work to ourselves, on the basis of our actual clinical needs. The Needs card is to knowledge management what your Goal card is to time management.

Both cards put you back in direct charge of your tools. But note this crucial difference: While you choose your own personal goal, what's on your Needs card is dictated by the necessities of your daily practice.

If you find yourself consistently turned off by what turns up on your Needs card, it may possibly be time to consider a change. One former radiologist of my acquaintance began to be bored by keeping up with her own specialty, and found herself avidly reading the psychiatry journals instead. Today she's a psychiatry resident—and no longer bored.

Now let's analyze the traditional ways we all acquire clinical knowledge, to see if they're maximally productive.

## Browsing the Journals

Surveys indicate that over 80% of physicians get new medical knowledge this way; the average doc spends about eight hours each month thumbing through journals.[2] Almost all of us have a pile of unread or half-read journals somewhere in our office, waiting for those spare moments when we can catch up on our reading. Of course, we never do quite catch up, because every month another bunch of new journals fattens our pile.

> ❝Although we may retain information we read long enough to pass a test, this kind of learning rarely results in changes in practice that lead to better patient care.❞
>
> Allen F. Shaughnessy, PharmD
> David C. Slawson, MD[3(p.2,157)]

Browsing journals and newsletters is an enjoyable activity; there's a familiar comfort in hanging out with all that information, and in just letting our natural curiosity and intellect have their head. But can we still afford to spend our limited CME time this way?

Think about it: If you browse the journals, what are the actual odds that a given journal article that you happen upon today (by random chance), will impact on a patient you may see (by random chance) soon enough for you to still recall (by random chance) what you learned, and apply it? That's too many random chances—the odds are almost zero. And knowledge that is not used quickly and repeatedly disappears back into the thundering background noise of the information explosion in a very short time.

So if you're just browsing the journals now without some kind of method, the best you can hope for is that by sheer serendipity and an awful lot of reading you'll run into something useful. Occasionally this does happen, and our browsing habit gets reinforced. But does that kind of random-walk medical education sound maximally effective and productive?

In a new study, 28 generalists were found to use journals to answer clinical questions about patients, as they actually came up in real time, in only 3% of cases. In over 50% of cases, they used desktop references.[4(p.1,513)] So why not convert your journals from an unusable, unruly pile to a handy desktop reference?

### "Surf and Turf" Your Journal Piles: Creating Your Own Customized Desktop Reference

In fact, this is what many physicians do. Here are some suggestions for getting through more journals in less time, while creating your own customized desktop reference, resulting in better retention and more efficient use of the new knowledge. As with paperwork, it comes down to having a method—and sticking to it.

1. First of all, you can **skip 50% of the papers** in most journals; they were not meant for you to read.

Most medical journals are published for two audiences: practicing docs (that's you) and researchers/academic physicians. About 50% of papers are by researchers just announcing to other researchers and academics the progress of important projects. There's tremendous pressure on academic researchers to publish or perish, but that doesn't mean you should feel any pressure to spend your valuable learning time reading all their stuff.

Another class of article you can probably ignore: any paper with a highly specialized focus, that doesn't connect at all to your existing knowledge base (this type of knowledge is represented by Point "O" in Figure 7–4). Say, for instance, you treat patients emergently if they're having a suspected MI, but you always get them quickly to an ER. You may find yourself nodding over an article on some complex aspects of EKG interpretation in acute MI—because at this point you just don't have enough knowledge about reading EKG's to connect the new information with. Studies show it's much harder to learn information or procedures that don't connect with your current knowledge base. (If you did some systematic review of EKG interpretation first, you could probably go back to the article and profit from it.)

Articles on the rarest, most trivial, and most obscure conditions, overspecialized topics far outside your practice, or researcher-to-researcher communications are of low utility to the busy practitioner with barely enough time to read at all. Skip them. You have more than enough on your plate just reading and absorbing the information that will be useful to you in your daily work.

2. As a matter of fact, you may be able to **throw out half your journals** for the same reasons. (Don't really throw them out; give them to your local medical librarian, or to someone who's sending journals to medical schools in disadvantaged areas of the world.) Keep those journals and magazines that cater directly to you, the practicing clinician. You'll still have too much to read

and absorb thoroughly, believe me—over 4,000 new journal articles appear *every day*.

3. Next, **stop trying to read your way through articles from beginning to end**. This is a tidal wave of information we're facing, my friend—if we don't surf it, we'll drown in it.

Where is it written you have to read books, journals, or papers from beginning to end? When you turn on your TV, do you stay on one channel from the beginning of the evening to sign-off? Never. To avoid all the commercials and other useless stuff, and find what is of personal interest to you, you generally scan, skim, skip, and switch around. You surf it.

Much of what's printed in journals may be very dear to the authors, but to you it's pure boilerplate. Do you really need to know the repetitive details of how ethical the researchers were, how many ANOVAS or logistical regressions they performed, etc., etc.? You're interested in the meat of the article: whether and how it's going to help you in your daily practice. Some academics keep insisting that we do our own sophisticated evaluations of research design, statistical methods, and the like. But that's their work—if we do it for them, will they see our patients for us? As someone who referees clinical research papers for a leading journal, I can assure you that it's the editors' responsibility to make sure their authors have used research methods which are honest and accurate. You don't have the time or the expertise to do the editor's work, either. If a journal publishes questionable stuff, and you have to pore over it to figure out if the work is authentic, stop reading that journal.

An example of how much excess (for us) detail there is in most journal articles: a recent paper on aspirin and fibrinolytic therapy for MI, published in a first-rank journal, ran to 14 pages and 97 references. Almost all of it comprised lengthy discussions of research methods and statistics. Only one half page was labeled "Implications for Clinical Practice."

> ❝You ask [experts] the time and they will tell you how to build a clock.❞
>
> Richard S. Wurman[5(p.125)]

So you can get through your journals at least twice as fast if you **surf, skim, scan, skip, speed-read**, etc. Process your journals when you're not going to be interrupted; scan the title, then the last few words of the abstract (giving you the conclusions). This should be enough to tell you whether you want the paper. (If you're in an electronic database, abstracts will have subject words lit up in the text to speed scanning.)

4. Think beyond what the journal's editor thinks everyone ought to be reading this month, and instead zone in on your unique personal needs. That's what your Needs card is for. **Use your Needs card as a guide while you're skimming.** Seek, clip, and save articles and reviews about whatever is on your card. If you've found a thin spot in your practical knowledge, and if a recent journal has a decent article on it, you've hit pay dirt.

5. To multiply your speed and breadth of coverage by another 200%, **put together a knowledge network** with three or four other professionals in your field. Each of you can skim three or four different journals a month, and clip useful articles to photocopy and send around the network. Make sure the other people in your network have a recent summary of your Needs card, and you have theirs. Now you have ten journals in your field covered every month, instead of four or five.

6. While reading and skimming quickly, note the most excellent articles, reviews, and updates that actually impact on the needs of your practice, as indicated by your own experience, and especially by your Needs card; **rip them out** (photocopy them if you read library journals, or scan and save them to disk or dis-

kette, etc.). Get rid of all the rest—luckily, you have a big wastebasket. But if you don't have a medical library nearby, you'll probably want to store your back issues somewhere out of the way, for possible future reference.

> **"**There are few systems which provide doctors with information at the time when they would be most likely to learn from it—when they are faced by a patient with a difficulty that could be satisfactorily solved.**"**
>
> —J.A.M. Gray[6(p.447)]

7. Now your pile of unread stuff should be down to about 1/20th of what it was. Here's the last step: **Don't (necessarily) read it.**

Instead, **file all of it in two folders** (or download it to your PC's database)—one marked "Workup" and the other, "Treatment." Add relevant parts of handouts from workshops and seminars that fit your needs. **Keep those two files on your desk** right in front of you where you will see them several times a day. (Clear away the other stuff—except your file of forms for dictating—to make room.)

Of course you may want to skim your two files from time to time so you know what's in them, and where to find something quickly when you need it. But the point is, you're not cramming for an exam that will be on a fixed date, and then will be over. Instead, you're creating a customized, flexible, continually updated personal knowledge base to be plugged into when you need it—your unique desktop reference.

### FOR HIGH-EFFICIENCY LEARNING IN THE TEACHABLE MOMENT, PULL ARTICLES OUT WHEN YOU NEED THEM

8. Now, whenever you have a case, question, or procedure which fits some of your filed articles, **pull the relevant articles**

**out** of the appropriate folder. If you have used your Needs card, this occasion may be just before the next visit of a patient whose case you found problematic.

You have now reached the teachable moment, and you have at hand everything you need for maximally efficient acquisition of new knowledge: the patient who needs your help, the preselected relevant and current information, and the personal motivation to learn it and use it.

So this is the ideal time to **study your materials very carefully**, underlining and annotating them as needed.

Take some time at this point (if you're managing your schedule better, you'll have the time) to **think about what you're reading** and how it relates to your case (or doesn't—not everything in print is accurate and complete).

### DON'T FORGET UNLEARNING

9. Now is also the time to **dump any outdated ideas** you may have had about how to evaluate and manage this type of case.

*Attitude alert:* Unlearning can be harder than learning new ways. Old ideas settle down to the bottom of your mind and stay there; it's a case of mental permafrost, "first in, last out." Some teachers assume that unlearning is automatic; good teachers know it is not.

Unlearning an Old Saw

A clever lecturer was trying to get physicians in his audiences to give up the overlearned but outdated aphorism, "Systolic blood pressure should be equal to age plus 100" (it should not). No matter how hard he tried, physicians held fast to the old saw.

Finally, he invented and taught a new aphorism: "If you believe systolic blood pressure is equal to age plus 100, your clinical IQ is equal to your age *minus* 100."

> This works like a charm. Every time the old saw comes up, the new one automatically kicks in and neutralizes it, making way for new knowledge.

The point is, you have to make a conscious effort to dump useless and outdated knowledge. It will also help if every now and then (but at least twice a year), you go through your two files and **throw out everything that's more than four years old**.

Using these nine suggestions, you'll quickly get rid of those guilt-inducing stacks of journals. In their place, you'll have exactly the streamlined, customized, updated knowledge you need most for your personal type of practice, at exactly the time and place you need it—so you can learn and apply the new knowledge dozens of times more efficiently than if you were just to go on browsing the journals randomly. If you use new knowledge in your practice right when you learn it, it "burns in" to your brain a lot deeper, and you're less likely to forget it.

---

Learning is not complete until you have put the new knowledge to work in your practice.

---

Exactly how you accumulate and store your personal knowledge base is up to you. Instead of (or in addition to) hard copy journals, you may prefer an off-the-shelf personal computerized database ("Pro-Cite" has been mentioned)—or one of your own devising. Any method of storage that works for you is excellent—don't let anyone bully you into feeling you have to use a computer, if that doesn't work for you.

You have only a limited amount of storage space for on-demand knowledge resources on your desk (or on your disk), and even less in your brain. The guiding principle is to make sure that what you're storing in both places is current, applicable to your unique practice, and instantly accessible when and where you need it. If your method fits these criteria, it's fine.

This all may sound a bit heretical, and may go against your ingrained habit—but more likely you're already using some method like the one described above to get through your journals. If not, consider the suggestions, see if they fit your personal learning style (more on this later), and, if they don't, make up your own method.

If you randomly browse journals to keep up with general medical and surgical knowledge, consider using medical news web sites (www.ama-assn.org gives advance journal article summaries), radio talk shows (the first 15 minutes of Dean Edell), or services like Johns Hopkins' "InteliHealth Professional Connect" (www.intelihealth.com), which will e-mail you news blurbs every day, with some ads and hype for Hopkins. You'll get the information a day or two earlier.

## Using Lectures and Tapes More Efficiently

About 80% of us also attend lectures with some regularity or use educational tapes.[7]

Compared with reading, getting information from a lecture may be slow; you're reading this book at about 300 words per minute, while the average speaker goes at half that speed. But the big problem with lectures and tapes is the same as with journals: How do we find, at exactly the right time, the right lecturer, teaching exactly the right subject, taught at our level, which we need right now for managing patients in our unique practice?

Many physicians habitually attend grand rounds or a department lecture every week or so, innocently trusting that what's being talked about will somehow be targeted to their current, unique learning needs, and that the presenter will be an effective teacher. Neither of these conditions is highly likely.

Here are a few suggestions for improving the odds of getting really useful personal knowledge from presentations:

1. **Give your input regularly to the CME committee of your staff, group, or association.** To be accredited, they're required to tailor programs to the actual needs of their physicians. Usually they'll welcome your input, since they want to arrange programs that fill your needs (and often they're out of ideas, anyway). Might as well **join your CME committee**, so you can do this on a regular basis; it usually doesn't meet too often.

2. **Send/bring the CME committee a summary of your Needs card** and ask them point blank to arrange the CME you need.

3. **Tell your CME committee if you've heard a good speaker or read a useful paper**—they may be able to get the speaker/author to come and give a presentation.

4. **Make sure your CME chair briefs all speakers thoroughly** about what you really need to know. Presenters at large medical association meetings these days get an average $2,000 a pop, plus expenses. Most of that comes out of your dues and registration, so get your money's worth: Demand that speakers meet your personal educational requirements.

CME program chairs routinely ask presenters to tailor their talks to the physician group they're speaking to, but speakers routinely resist, feeling that they're the experts and already know exactly what audiences need to learn. I've walked out of some snoozingly boring talks by presenters who had not taken the trouble to check with our CME chair to find out their audience's level of expertise and interest. As a result, the lecture had nothing to do with the kind of patients we see, or was pitched below our existing knowledge level. The *ars* is much too *longa* and the *vita* much too *breva* for us to be sitting through useless lectures, just out of politeness or inertia. Walk.

5. Some presenters are excellent at researching, organizing, cooking down, and presenting useful clinical materials in such a way that it all makes sense to the audience, and sticks with them. A star teacher can give you more unforgettable and useful pearls in 20 minutes of aphorisms and anecdotes than a 200-slide wonder-boy can in two hours. It almost doesn't matter what the subject is (as long as they're experienced in it)—you learn faster from these people. **If you find a star teacher** in your field, you've found gold. **Get maximum exposure** to him: Go to more of his presentations, order his tapes, and arrange for him to speak more often at meetings you attend. After a while, your own expertise may grow to a point where you don't get as much from his lectures; it's time to look for a new teacher with new pearls.

6. **Try to attend meetings of organizations that take the trouble to customize their programs** so they're of real practical value to you.

Sometimes we attend a CME conference because it's being held in a warm spot with palm trees, and not because of the educational value of the program. Nothing wrong with that—rest and relaxation are good for us—but if we're not selective about what conferences we attend, we can easily end up at Point "O" on our knowledge diagram in Figure 7–4.

Recently an internist friend signed up for a conference in a coastal resort. Frankly, it wasn't his first choice for educational value, but he wanted the break. Once there, he found himself in an advanced lecture on the intricacies of examining the foot. He had never imagined there were so many dozens of things you could do to a foot...totally fascinating!

But also useless for my friend, who never does such complicated foot exams; he always calls the local orthopod, an expert. Since the program chair of this particular conference had thrown him a curve (it was advertised as an internal medicine seminar), my friend exited the hall to enjoy the fresh ocean air.

In the past five years, most associations have been changing their programs to be more practitioner focused. Magazines catering to medical meeting planners run many articles urging them to offer practical courses that address our real problems. Stick with associations that actually do this. Also, look for longer meetings. Some research suggests that short CME meetings (less than a day) are not as effective as longer conferences.[8]

Even if you can't find the perfect meeting, go to some meeting every year anyway...and enjoy the fresh air and the palm trees. That will be good for your productivity, too.

### The Most Popular CME May Be the Least Useful

Now for the surprise punch line: Browsing the journals and passively listening to lectures—though by far the most popular educational activities—are, for most of us, the *least* effective ways of changing the way we practice. In fact, several studies have indicated that reading and audiovisual programs both failed to produce much measurable change in physicians' practice patterns.[9]

So why do we keep on browsing and listening? Because it's easy, familiar, comfortable, and handy. But still not very effective.

Of course, if you have the time and inclination to read through all your journals cover to cover, and to attend whatever lectures and seminars are routinely scheduled—and if this is your conscious choice and if this works for you—then don't change.

What you actually do to keep up your clinical skills isn't crucial; the crucial change you do want to make is in your own attitude toward your continuing professional education. Realize that you can no longer afford to be the passive recipient of what someone else has guessed you need to learn. Take an active, aggressive, informed role in getting yourself the best training available to meet the current needs of your unique practice.

Just as college professors argue endlessly over "the canon" (what books should be taught), medical educators have for many decades been contending over what should or should not be in the medical curriculum. The actual truth: It's not the curriculum that makes a good physician—it's the student.

How well you will be trained in the coming years is really not up to the professors; it's up to you.

Now let's move on to consider using other methods of knowledge management that may be more efficient than browsing journals and passively attending lectures.

---

**Notes**

1. J.C. Sibley et al., "A Randomized Trial of Continuing Medical Education," *The New England Journal of Medicine* 306 (1982): 511–515.
2. D. Erickson, "CME Notes," *Medical Meetings,* December 1997, 9.
3. A. Shaughnessy and D. Slawson, "Getting the Most from Review Articles," *American Family Physician* 55, no. 6 (1997): 2,155–2,160.
4. A. Barrie and A. Ward, "Questioning Behavior in General Practice," *British Medical Journal* 315 (1997): 1,512–1,515.
5. R.S. Wurman, *Information Anxiety* (New York: Bantam, 1990).
6. J.A.M. Gray, "Continuing Education—Which Techniques Are Effective?" *Lancet,* 23 August, 1980, 447–448.
7. Erickson, *Medical Meetings,* 9.
8. D.A. Davis et al., "Changing Physician Performance," *Journal of the American Medical Association* 274 (1995): 700–705.
9. Davis et al., *Journal of the American Medical Association,* 702.

## ✦ 9 ✦

# "See One, Do One, Screw One": How to Learn Faster

We practicing physicians use several sources to maintain and update our personal clinical knowledge base, including:

- ✦ our own clinical experience (including our errors)
- ✦ other physicians
- ✦ our patients
- ✦ co-workers (nurses, pharmacists, et al.)
- ✦ thinking, talking, teaching, and writing about our work
- ✦ reading books and journals
- ✦ formal educational activities such as lectures and courses
- ✦ electronic databases and online resources

We've already suggested some methods for getting more out of reading, lectures, and tapes, and we've noted that passive reading and listening may actually be, for many of us, the least efficient ways of getting useful knowledge. Also, the type of knowledge we can get from published textbooks and articles, and from most lectures and electronic databases, is general and statistical. Often that's not the kind of knowledge we require; we need specific guidance in how we should proceed in the case of a unique, individual patient. Pre-packaged knowledge bases of all kinds simply are not efficient sources for this kind of guidance.

So we have to pick up a lot of our useful clinical knowledge outside formal educational experiences, while we're on the fly, working with patients and colleagues. This important process, used daily by every practicing physician, is ignored when academics discuss continuing medical education. Let's look at how we might make it more efficient.

### Your Personal Panel of Experts

Going in, one tenet of our education needs to be re-examined in the face of the explosion in medical knowledge: *No one of us can know everything we need to know anymore,* and we shouldn't be ashamed to admit it—as long as we know who knows what we don't know, and how to get hold of them fast.

In medical school we were expected to know the answer to everything we were asked. If we'd ever said to a professor, "Well, sir...I personally don't know the answer, but my classmate here is pretty solid in that area, so if you'll excuse me, I'll just ask him, and get right back to you"—forget it, we'd have been outta there before we could finish the sentence.

It doesn't make practical sense for every one of us to try to become expert in everything. Getting heavy experience (which is what makes you an expert) in so many different areas is impossible. Better to spend your time becoming truly excellent at what you do best and most often—and **set up a personal panel of experts** for delivering other specialized clinical knowledge, when and where you need it. The time which you save by consulting these experts can be applied to other tasks.

But this works for everyone involved only if you **keep up your end by maximizing your personal expertise in your own field**. It's your unstated duty to the other docs on your personal panel to acquire new knowledge and methods, apply them in your own practice, and share what you learn.

For example, an internist friend in New England has a busy hospital-based practice in complicated geriatric cases. Like most practitioners, he spends time on the phone or in the corridor getting curbside consults, quick reality checks, and mini-educational updates from several other medical, surgical, and psychiatric specialists and subspecialists. They know more than he does about how to handle various specialized problems that come up in the cases he sees. He realizes he could never run his practice without their expert knowledge and experience.

In return, they call him when they need advice in his area of expertise, and he always gives it freely (or tells them someone else they can call). He says he's flattered that they consider him a resource; probably, each colleague on his personal panel is also pleased that he holds them enough above their peers to call them first for help. He also sends them a lot of formal consults, and they tend to schedule his patients very promptly.

To the extent that your health plan contracts allow, you probably already have arrangements of this sort in your own medical community. You may also have discovered that it pays to have two people on your panel in key specialties, in case you can't reach one of them. One more advantage of being in close touch with a panel of excellent physicians is that when the time comes for you to join a group, change your group, or form a group, you already know where to start: with your panel of experts.

Just two caveats about having your own panel: Professionals not on it may feel left out, and their egos may be bruised (which is not a minor injury). Say you phone Dr. A, your curbside consultant of choice, and the receptionist says Dr. A is out, but would you like to talk to his partner, Dr. B? Don't say, "No, I need to talk to someone with brains." (This actually happened to a colleague.)

Also, dumping your patient late at night or on a weekend, so that the on-call specialist will have to see her, is not a courteous way to practice medicine. Getting curbside consults and second opinions is something we all do; you don't need to be sneaky about it. Make the request yourself.

## Your Personal Knowledge Network

In addition to this personal panel of expert consultants, my internist friend also consciously networks with two or three first-rate professionals whose knowledge base touches but does not duplicate his own. They excel in corners of his specialty that he doesn't have enough formal training and experience in to be an expert (one is a knowledgeable pharmacist, because my friend runs into a lot of thorny problems in differential therapeutics and multiple drug interactions among his elderly patients).

He knows how to get hold of these three professionals fast (within an hour or less), and is in touch with them at least once or twice every week, sometimes even daily. Over the years, he's been extremely careful to cultivate their friendship and trust—which is easy, because he admires their work a great deal. He returns their phone calls before others', and thinks they return his first, too.

My friend also "stores" clinical information in his knowledge network. When he comes across a useful article or tape, he circulates a copy of it to his network. Later, if he has lost track of that information himself, he can ask one of them, and they'll often have the information he needs.

Thus, he gets and gives expert knowledge that effectively expands the collective knowledge base of his entire informal panel and network, and everyone's patients get a higher level of care than any single practitioner could hope to offer. It's a win-win-win.

By extending your knowledge base this way, you have the expertise of several skilled practitioners literally at your fingertips, and they can probably answer the frequently asked questions that are so hard to access in the literature, even by computer: What's the prognosis of this individual patient? What's the natural history of this illness? Which of the many treatments available for this illness best fits this individual case? Is this symptom ever seen in this illness, or should I start looking for a second diagnosis to explain it? etc.

Understand going in that your personal *knowledge network* will be different from your *group* (the doctors you're in business with), your *team* (the professionals you work side by side with), and your *crew* (all the people in your specialty who work in one location). Your personal network is chosen and maintained by you, and serves the specific purpose of enhancing your personal efficiency and accuracy.

Networking is a highly developed skill in other professions and in management, where it replaces disappearing centralized hierarchies and lines of command. As our practices also shift away from hospitals and their corridors crowded with colleagues, we physicians need to be a little less shy about setting up intentional professional networks outside our usual groups and teams. Our mutually shared knowledge, experience, and devotion to getting the best care for our patients make us natural networkers. Also, in medicine we still have a great tradition of sharing knowledge freely, for the good of our patients. Finally, at least one recent study shows that physicians doing research who have more extensive colleague networks are more productive.[1]

Now it's just a question of doing it.

 **Exercise 9–1** Take a minute to reflect on what condition your personal knowledge network is in. Could it use a tune-up? List on an index card the names (and phone numbers) of the three or four colleagues you consult with most frequently. Keep the card with you, and decide over time whether you need to add or drop names.

Do you sometimes go for days or weeks without talking at length with another doc? Try to **cultivate your**

**network**, beyond the sharing of clinical knowledge. Coffee and lunches; phone calls; and the occasional book, software, or other small gift are all appropriate. The more you put into your network, the more it will give back to you.

## Look at Others' Errors

Although it's not a very reassuring thing to harp on with patients, we physicians actually do **learn from errors**, perhaps even more than we do from cases that are error free.

Popular medical journals have begun recently to print case reports containing clinical errors, in the hopes that if we can read about—and recognize—others' clinical errors, maybe we can avoid making the same errors ourselves. This seems a valid approach to more efficient learning.[2]

> ❝Give me a fruitful error any time, full of seeds, bursting with its own corrections!❞
>
> Wilfred Pareto

Physicians have suggested that if you **sit on your medical staff peer review committee**, you can get a crash course in clinical errors—and, hopefully, error reduction. The errors being made by other docs in your own medical community are particularly apt for you to hear and think about. Peer review is one of the few places in all of medicine where it's not only OK to talk about physician errors, it's pretty much all you'll do.

At your first committee meeting, after a few silent gasps of, "There but for the grace of God go I," you'll likely vow to begin quietly updating your personal knowledge base in areas where your peers are dropping the ball, and where you realize you could use some brushing up yourself. If you **take your Needs card to peer review committee meetings**, you can unobtrusively jot down these recognized needs for future follow-up.

## Learn from Your Own Errors

We can learn more efficiently from our own errors by taking two steps.

First, we don't need to wait for major errors to happen before we start learning. They're too uncommon (thank the Lord!) to give us a meaningful sample, and we obviously would prefer to catch our own patterns of deficiency before any patient is hurt, and before any peer review is involved. Informal studies of physician errors show that we practitioners routinely make "near misses"— small errors that either have no clinical significance, or are caught and neutralized by ourselves, someone else, or by a fail-safe built into our delivery system.

For example, if you're prescribing a statin for a hypercholesterolemic patient and then add niacin, you may get a computer-screen flag or a call from the pharmacy alerting you that, if given together, the two drugs can cause liver damage. You may decide it's not worth the risk, and cancel the niacin. No harm done.

But if you realize this was a near miss, you'll add to your Needs card: "Interactions with statins." If you're alert, you may catch as many as one or two near misses like this a month; that kind of volume, over the years, can guide you to where you need to brush up or get further targeted training. So, **analyze your near misses** by noting down every one of them on a separate card (don't label this card) and looking for patterns of deficient attention, skill, or knowledge that you can remedy.

> Zaslove's Law: If you find one error or slip in a case, always search painstakingly for others in the same case; you'll usually find them.

Studies of clinical errors also suggest that docs seem to gain if we can **discuss clinical errors with another practitioner**. Not only does this give us psychological relief, it also has benefits in increasing the knowledge base of both practitioners. And we can discuss a lot besides errors.

## We Need to Talk!

It seems that the simple act of talking about something has an effect on brain metabolism, and definitely speeds knowledge acquisition. To **regularly discuss your clinical work** is a super-efficient way of learning because:

✦ it's case driven, so you're hooking up knowledge to your practical clinical needs
✦ it's interactive (with a human, not a software program); instead of just memorizing lists and protocols, when you discuss a case you're retrieving old knowledge and rehearsing its application in your (and your colleague's) cases
✦ it's emotionally meaningful and a pleasant social experience
✦ it puts you in touch with all the clinical knowledge, experience, judgment, wisdom, and intuition that another physician has accumulated. That physician, in turn, is in contact with other people in the wider medical community, and so

on—you're actually plugged into a living network of in-depth information that makes the Internet seem thin by comparison.

Cognitive psychology has established that hooking up knowledge and experience to practical needs and to preexisting knowledge, retrieving knowledge and rehearsing its use, and adding meaning and emotion to knowledge are all terrific ways to enhance the learning process. When you discuss your cases with someone, you're automatically and painlessly doing all of those things; so this can be a much more efficient way of learning than passive exposure to the same materials.

### Keep in Touch—Or Get Blown Away

This winter I took off a few days and drove to the desert to work on this book. One morning it seemed unusually windy, but there were no bulletins on the radio, so I set off for a scenic drive that a friend had recommended.

Fortunately, I stopped for coffee on the way, and fell into conversation with a local. When I told him where I was headed, he told me that my planned drive would be very dangerous—if I could make it at all. "The highways out of town are closed because there's sand blowing 70 miles an hour," he said. "And unless you cover 'em with Saran wrap, you'll end up with your car windows sandblasted solid."

I paid the check and drove straight back to my motel, impressed once again with how important it is to keep in constant touch with the people around you.

## So Who Can You Talk To?

From consultants and experts in your knowledge network, you'll get just-in-time opinions about pressing clinical questions, and they'll also alert you to new wrinkles (for example, a not-yet-reported side effect of a brand-new medication).

But you'll also benefit enormously if you can **find one colleague–friend with whom you can regularly discuss your clinical work in depth**. Sit down face to face over coffee or a sandwich (the phone's OK sometimes) with this person for a half hour or so every few days, or as often as makes sense, to discuss one or two of your cases—with total frankness.

But to do this, you need to find one physician in your field who will understand your patients and your type of practice, listen sympathetically and not criticize you in a negative way, and give you expert advice without being obnoxious about it.

It's probably better if your confidant does not work in your group, and does not work side by side with you in your team. (It turns out that if you share responsibilities for some of the same cases, each of you tends to be invested in being "right" about how to handle a given case, and that kind of strongly defended opinion isn't what's needed for efficient two-way learning.)

So you're generally better off with someone outside your group and your team, who has a similar practice (but not so similar that you're in competition). Why not pick the top doc in your medical community to buddy with? He could use a friend, too, I assure you. Just make sure it's someone who'll freely give you honest feedback in a positive way, and who'll offer creative suggestions about your clinical work in a spirit of mutual respect and collegial friendship—with a little humor and irony thrown in.

Sound more like a saint than a physician? How do you find a colleague like this?

There's only one way: You yourself need to be that kind of "peer pal" for someone else. No one gives you this kind of invaluable service unless you freely give them the same in return. But an arrangement like this is priceless, and your friend (you'll inevitably become friends) is bound to recognize quickly how valuable this arrangement is for him, also.

Not only can you both go deeply into your cases—especially those most valuable of all, the ones where you may have made an error in judgment—but you also get to hear in detail how someone else at your level handles their thorniest cases, and to make suggestions. You'll gain knowledge from both sides of the experience.

And this is not even to mention the 100% support and acceptance, the expert shoulder to cry on, and the camaraderie that you enjoy as a perk in such a collegial friendship; these boost your morale enormously, when you need it most. Everyone has some bad days, when doubt and discouragement make you drag; call your friend, talk it out, and you're back for more.

Without realizing it, we physicians can become lonely in our professional lives. Isolated from intimate, friendly contact with colleagues at our level, and preoccupied with our problems and responsibilities, we can lose perspective, become depressed, and miss the spice of doctoring—and not even know why. Because of the new pressures and insecurities of practice, the splintering of professional roles, etc., this is happening to more and more of us.

As physicians, we feel a personal imperative to work and be productive at our art; as humans, we have a powerful instinct to be socially intimate and share our experiences; a close peer friendship lets us satisfy both. So if you don't have such a relationship now, I highly recommend that you start looking around for one, then cultivate it carefully and steadily, day by day, over the years. It can help you become more knowledgeable, more productive— and much happier.

P.S.: Don't be overly exclusive in your peer friendship. If other docs in your medical community feel you two are snooting them, they can get annoyed with you.

## Exams, Presenting, and Other Stuff We Hate

If passively browsing journals and listening to lectures are not the most efficient means of structured learning for most of us, what methods are better?

Look over the next checklist. You'll recognize most of the methods—from medical school and residency!

If your heart sinks or your palms sweat when you look over these suggestions, don't worry. It's true that once we're safely out of training and busy in practice, we naturally tend to avoid doing any of these things—yet they are probably some of the fastest, surest, and most efficient methods we can use to acquire new clinical knowledge. (Which is why they made us use them in medical school and residency in the first place.)

So to use our limited CME time most efficiently, we have to bite the bullet and do some things that require more effort. However, we can now take control, reshape them to fit our busy lives, and ensure that the knowledge we're acquiring is appropriate to our needs. Luckily, there are some ways we can do these things efficiently, without becoming too uncomfortable, and we'll stress these user-friendly methods for mature practitioners. If we actually do some of them regularly, they'll become comfortable habits again, also.

1. **Take exams.** Most journals and throwaway clinical letters now include little quizzes and self-tests you can take to see if you've retained the information; quizzes are available online and on many instructional CD-ROMs, also.

Like the tests we took in school, though, these quizzes sometimes tend to stress annoying minutiae instead of useful clinical knowledge. Their main utility at our level is to make sure we are actually absorbing the materials. So rather than automatically skipping them, if you make it a habit to take (and score) them, your learning efficiency can go up a bit.

A phone call to a residency program near you will get you the latest qualifying exam or mock boards in your field. Some journals regularly run sample board exam questions, and you'll find books full of them at your medical center bookstore. Many educational CD-ROMs contain board-type questions; you can jump to the answers electronically.

If every few years you take mock board exams and score them yourself, you can spot where you need to update your fund of general knowledge in your field. Add that information to your Needs card.

2. **Get handbooks.** Reading the latest basic text in your field from cover to cover is probably not your idea of an exciting weekend. For one thing, general textbooks tend to be somewhat out of date because of the publishing time lag. They focus on disease entities and pathology, and are a little sketchy on the patient-centered approach we need. Also, since they usually discuss only prototypical cases, these books may seem bland or oversimplified to experienced practitioners.

But quickly skim-reading a new text in your field every four or five years gives you a broader view of where things fit together, catches you up on wrinkles you may have missed, and tips you off if you're inadvertently avoiding a whole chunk of your specialty. Keeping the latest texts (paperback ones are cheap) in your office lets you review a discrete area of clinical information when your Needs card dictates; there are usually lists of good review articles, though not very recent ones (a quicker way to get recent review articles is by accessing www.CME-reviews.com).

If you don't already have them, also consider getting recent paperback handbooks of the specialties closest to yours (I keep neurology and internal medicine) for your office shelf, and annotate or sticker what you use most often. Brushing up quickly just before you call a consultant lets you ask the right questions—in fact, you may not need to call at all.

3. **Give a lecture.** Preparing a lecture for your nursing or office staff on some clinical topic that comes up frequently is a painless way of starting to teach, and has added dividends:

- ✦ mutual respect (you may be surprised at how much specialized knowledge about your field they already have)
- ✦ a better understanding, on both sides, of why you do certain procedures, have certain priorities, etc.
- ✦ a prestige example for your staff, who will then start doing more cross-training with each other, increasing their efficiency
- ✦ you'll be amazed at how much organizing and deep thinking about your personal knowledge base you'll do to prepare even a simple subject in a thorough, systematic way.

4. Ditto for **presenting** at case conferences and grand rounds. Don't worry about humiliating yourself by revealing some huge gap in your clinical knowledge in front of your peers. In years of speaking before dozens of audiences made up of distinguished medical and surgical practitioners much more capable than myself, I've found that practicing physicians really respect the effort you're making, and always graciously overlook your gaffes. After all, you're a fellow-practitioner, not a professor, and at least you had the guts to get up there. Meanwhile, out of sheer survival instinct, you're sure to become much more familiar with whatever it is you're presenting—and from then on you'll be considered a resource by your colleagues.

5. **Do a Mini-Residency.** University teaching hospitals and clinics really do have stunningly high standards of care and use the newest approaches for a wide array of challenging cases. Besides the knowledge you pick up by listening and watching and asking questions, and the benchmarking you can do to ensure that your own practice is cutting-edge, you learn a lot just by osmosis. It's wisely said, "If you sit next to a block of ice you automatically get

cold." There's more to practicing than just knowledge: Watching excellent physicians as they make clinical decisions can subtly but definitely improve your own methods of decision making—this can be more valuable than new knowledge. Try if possible to go on real bedside rounds, so you can watch (and demonstrate) history taking and examinations on real patients.

Periodically hanging out with very smart people has a stimulating effect on us intellectually; it's also inspiring to be with physicians who are dedicated to excellence, and who remind us of what a high calling we're in.

Maybe you think you'll be looked down on by the high-powered university-based knowledge transmitters, but my experience has been the opposite: They respect the level of skill we busy practitioners achieve by dint of the sheer volume of cases we handle. A friend of mine recently asked a professor of ophthalmology whether he considered himself the best qualified person to do a certain procedure. The professor's answer: "No, I spend too much of my time on teaching and research, so I don't really have the volume of procedures to be the best. There's a fellow on the Coast who does hundreds of these every year, and nothing else—he's probably tops in the country."

6. **Do Research.** No matter what you've been led to believe, you don't need a grant or a university appointment to do useful clinical research. A sharp eye and some curiosity about the patients you see are sufficient. You can sign up with one of the huge multi-practice studies that are getting under way now, or you can follow your own lead.

Observational studies can be as valuable to other practitioners as massive controlled trials, and in fact, most big trials are designed to test the observations of some busy clinician like you. Several years ago I observed that a couple of patients on Thorazine had developed definite signs of a B vitamin deficiency. One Saturday afternoon at the library yielded the information that this had been noticed in rats, but never reported in humans. A few months later my paper on it was published, and now there are several confirmatory papers in the literature from university research centers.[3]

### Discovery from Down Under

Barry J. Marshall was an Australian internist who, in 1980, first discovered the connection between peptic ulcer disease and infection with *H. pylori*. He was young and unknown, and he lived far from the huge medical centers where ulcer disease was known definitely to be related to stress and acid production—not to bacterial infection.

To prove he was correct, the young practitioner swallowed some of the bacterium himself—and developed gastritis. Though his discovery was greeted with skepticism and attacked publicly by established academic researchers, Marshall had one advantage: He was right. Finally, in 1992, his work was confirmed, and is now accepted.

The young internist changed the way ulcer disease is treated in its over 500 million victims.[4]

So try doing some clinical research. The payoffs: You'll get really interested in your work in that area, learn in greater depth, add to the general fund of medical knowledge—and get lots of glory in the form of postcards from Albania requesting reprints of your paper.

## How to Learn a New Procedure Faster

With so many new or improved technologies, drug protocols, treatment modalities, and surgical techniques for physicians to learn how to use, there's been more pressure to discover how we can learn a new procedure in the shortest possible time. Here's a brief summary of what seems to work for many physicians:

1. **Commit yourself** psychologically to learning the new technique. We learned more quickly in school and training because we had to—i.e., we were fully committed. Decide going in that there will be no quitting.
2. If possible, **find a highly skilled practitioner to imitate**. Make sure she's someone who will slow down, explain the reasons for what she's doing, and take the time to critique you as she checks you out on the procedure. In other words, she should be not only a good technician, but also a good coach.
3. **Have training sessions in private** to avoid embarrassment, especially if you're rusty at basic technique. You don't need the extra sweat of performing for an audience.
4. **Grasp the sequential steps first by analyzing the procedure intellectually** (self-talk helps).
5. **Practice individual sub-units** of the procedure until you've fixed each one in your mind (chipping). Don't go on to another sub-unit until you've mastered the earlier one—you'll probably forget the first one, if you do this.
6. **Practice the whole procedure on your own over and over**, to gain speed, smoothness, and proficiency.
7. When you're ready, **use the new skills as soon and as often as possible** in your daily practice.
8. **Don't become discouraged by poor outcomes at first.** Most procedures take several (even several dozen) reps for basic proficiency, hundreds for mastery.
9. **Be prepared to work hard.** If it's been some years since you were in training, you may have forgotten the brain-sweat, curses, gritted teeth, and repeated failures of those years. Recognize the aphorism, "See three, try four, miss

them all!'"? One medical student team's wry motto was, "Our best is none too good."

Learning new procedures is long, hard, sometimes frustrating work. It's also very rewarding: You gain in mastery and self-confidence. Your patients get better care. When more of us get smarter sooner, our whole profession moves forward another giant step. That's a win-win-win.

And don't forget: "...teach one."

---

**Notes**

1. M. Hitchcock et al., "Professional Networks," *Academic Medicine* 70, no. 12 (1995): 1,108–1,116.
2. J. Brown et al., "Learning from Our Errors," *The New England Journal of Medicine* 335, no. 14 (1996): 1,049–1,053.
3. M. Zaslove, "Severe Ariboflavinosis," *Journal of Orthomolecular Psychiatry* 12, no. 2 (1983): 113–115.
4. A. Primrose and S. Katz, *Writing in the Sciences* (New York: St. Martins, 1998), 175–211.

# ✦ 10 ✦

# Do You Need a Computer to Keep Up?

No single technology will automatically make every physician more productive. It's also a bad idea to let any machine eat up our time or dominate our lives; they are our slaves, we are not theirs. I believe in taking charge of our machines, planting our foot firmly on their neck, and making the best (most sensible, humane) use of any technology that will meet our unique clinical needs. We shouldn't take any crap from people who pressurize us to buy or use their gadgets if we don't want or need them.

However, common sense tells us to take advantage of current technology if that's the only practical way to accomplish what we need to accomplish for our patients. Even if you're allergic to computers, you don't refuse to order CAT scans or cash checks because they're generated by computers. But we physicians have been slow to embrace electronic databases and networked personal computers in our daily clinical work.

Think about this: The acceleration of knowledge creation and dissemination in medicine is being powered by the explosion of information technology (networked computers; MEDLINE, the Web, and other online databases; fast electronic printing and copying; CD-ROMs; etc.). Taking advantage of this same technology to keep up with clinical knowledge not only makes sense, it has now become a necessity for achieving the highest efficiency in personal knowledge management.

In short, we need to use machines to keep up with the machines.

How many of us use personal computers in our daily clinical work? Depends on how you ask, who you ask, and what you're selling. A recent survey by a tech company said that 43% of physicians were using the Internet for "professional purposes."[1(p.21)] Yet a survey of g.p.'s found they were using online clinical databases to answer only 1% of questions during office hours (they mostly used desktop references and calls to colleagues).[2(p.1,513)] At a recent university-sponsored productivity seminar, I asked everyone who was regularly accessing MEDLINE (or other electronic databases) to raise their hands. I was shocked: Out of 100 specialists, fewer than 10 raised their hands.

The usual reasons docs give for not using personal computers in clinical work: "No time"; "I'm not trained"; "No access"; "My computer is out of date." But if you're already online, you'll probably agree that docs who are not accessing electronic clinical knowledge bases are missing a valuable aid to their work (and you'll want to skim over the next few pages); if you're not yet there, let me try to convince you of how much going online can increase your productivity.

### The "Killer App" for Docs

If there's any one "killer application"—that is, one reason why you *must* have ready access to electronic databases for clinical knowledge management—it's MEDLINE.

It doesn't matter whether you access MEDLINE via your own organization's intranet, an Internet service provider (ISP), or CD-ROM—as long as you do access it. This National Library of Medicine database contains eight million references and abstracts, accessible 24-seven by anyone anywhere in the world at the touch of a key. It can do things for your daily practice that there simply is no other way to do. It's pure gold.

### Searching 1,000 References in Four Seconds

A generalist wished to start a diabetic on one of the newer antidepressants, paroxetine (Paxil), for behavioral symptoms. She was unsure if there were any special precautions to observe in prescribing Paxil for patients with diabetes. The physician found no help in the PDR, and calls to her knowledge network and the drug company turned up nothing.

So the physician booted up her PC, went online to MEDLINE, and keyed in "paroxetine." She got over 1,000 entries. Then she keyed in "diabetes mellitus" and got 104,000 entries.

In the old days of hard-copy *Index Medicus,* she would have had to do a laborious hand search through as many as 1,000 papers for any that mentioned a relationship between paroxetine and DM; this would have taken weeks.

Instead, she pushed one button, and in four seconds she had on her screen the citation for the one paper out of over 100,000 that discussed DM and paroxetine.[3] She had hit pay dirt. She was able to find the paper in her hospital's medical library and manage her patient quickly and confidently.

That's a killer application.

Such high-speed utility makes electronic knowledge management as indispensable as your stethoscope. Up to this point I have avoided saying that electronic databases are indispensable to achieving maximum productivity. In this one area, they are.

> ❝Machines were made to work,
> and people to think.❞
>
> Old IBM slogan

### If You're a Cyberphobe, This One's for You

Doctors at productivity seminars let loose with a lot of frustration, impatience, and embarrassment when we get to the subject of personal computers. Surgeons who daily perform complex six-hour procedures confess they've tried to learn personal computing and have given up. Some docs say frankly they've stopped using their home computer; they can't stand being embarrassed by their children, who can run rings around them at the keyboard.

Since so few of us are using personal computers in our daily clinical decision making, I've included a step-by-step exercise sketching out a painless way to get connected. In San Diego, a seminar participant took the microphone to tell his fellow endoscopic surgeons that this one exercise was, in his opinion, the single most valuable change they could make in their practice. He felt that accessing online knowledge bases was that important for personal productivity.

 **Exercise 10–1 Use a Networked Personal Computer in Your Daily Clinical Work.**

1. Buy or lease your own machine (sharing machines is less productive). Decent desktops go for $1,500, laptops for twice that; excellent machines lease for

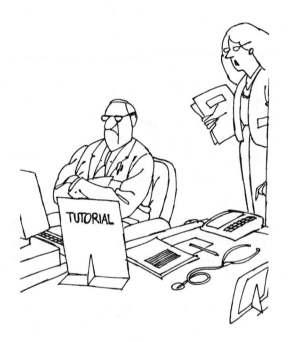

"…Would you like to take five and treat a patient or two?"

$70-$150 monthly (you can buy at the end of the lease for $1). If this sounds steep, understand that you're not paying for the gadget—you're paying for a 300,000,000-page database.

If you will use it in more than one location, consider a laptop; if you move around a lot, get one under six pounds. Faster chips and more memory, etc. are definitely better—you can do everything quicker—so get the "fastest with the mostest" that makes sense financially. You'll need a CD-ROM drive; a fast modem; some preinstalled basic software (all packaged with your machine); and a quiet, fast inkjet or laser printer (usually bought separately). Don't skimp on memory or processor speed—you will need it all to keep up with new applications.

2. Have your guru or your vendor set your desktop system up for you; they'll do it in hours, saving you days of frustration (laptops are more straightforward).

3. Word processing (using your computer as a smart typewriter) is not a stretch. You just load some software (Word or WordPerfect), get a simple book (the *"Dummies"* series is OK), and find someone to talk you through the early stages (a guru). *Warning:* Even such "simple" procedures as loading software can turn ugly. So *don't try to start computing without an on-call guru; it's too frustrating.*

4. Have all your computer training and practice sessions in private, far away from snickering office staff, colleagues, and your clinical duties. Under no circumstances let your kids instruct you! Allow sev-

eral sessions spread over weeks or months to learn the basics—computers are not user-friendly or intuitive; the ads lie. Hang in there, surrender to your computer, be humble. Yelling at it or hitting it will not help (I've tried both). At all times, while learning, resist the sudden strong impulses you will have to throw your computer out the window.

5. So far, this is no big deal; typing on a solitary computer isn't too exciting. But once you're comfortably using your computer as a typewriter, you can use your fax modem to transmit what you've typed.

6. Next, you can connect your machine to the biggest machine in the world: the worldwide network of 40,000,000 other computers, the Internet.

   The simplest possible way to the Net and the Web (the graphics part of the Net) is to activate some of the preloaded software on your computer to connect with an ISP. You could phone them, but their lines are always busy. For 10 or 20 bucks a month you'll get e-mail, access to the Net, the Web, and MEDLINE (and lots of obnoxious, unsolicited porn ads).

7. Now that you know how to get online, learn from your guru (or a course, book, journal article, or from your medical librarian) how to access and search MEDLINE. There are many routes; have your guru "bookmark" several of them so you never have to wait around to get in.

   It's definitely best to have someone talk you through your first few MEDLINE searches. Don't be frustrated or discouraged; it takes several searches over several weeks to get it. Use your Needs card as a guide to what you want to search for. You'll find most online citations have abstracts attached. Since there are only a few full-text journals online, you'll still need to xerox some journal articles in a library, send for reprints (slow), or have them faxed (expensive).

If you're religiously opposed to using a computer, **find someone who can do MEDLINE searches for you** (a medical librarian, a pharmacist, one of your office staff, etc.). This arrangement is not as good as personal access, but after a few weeks or months of having someone search MEDLINE for you, you'll realize how invaluable the database is, and you'll be more motivated to learn how to do it yourself.

You certainly can live without e-mail by using your phone, voice mail, and fax; and your secretary can do all your word processing. But there simply is no other, non-computerized way to access these clinical databases with even one one-thousandth of the speed and breadth available via computer. So I've made getting computerized a very strong suggestion. If you follow it, the world of electronic knowledge management will open up to you—you'll learn to do sophisticated, "gold standard" searches online; share your cases and questions in chat rooms, online journal clubs, and mailing lists (discussion groups); browse, search, visit, and download from medical web sites; etc.

### Don't Let Anyone Put You Off or Discourage You

Unfortunately, some of the people who are already online and accessing these information resources like to annoy people who aren't doing it yet—"What? I can't believe you're not wired! You mean you actually don't go up to the chronic myeloproliferative disease web site every hour? You're missing so much" (i.e., you're hopelessly out of date and a dud, probably an inferior person).

Ignore these people. By being so obnoxious about their computer prowess, they discourage physicians like you from getting started. Don't let them scare you away from an indispensable tool with their smart-ass jargon about aperture-grill CRTs and raster outputs; you definitely won't need to know any of that crap to get what you need from a computer. To clear up all the mystery: Clinicians basically use computers for word processing, e-mail, and accessing clinical databases. Beyond these, sitting and staring at a screen for hours every day is not really productive.

So go for it. You're plenty smart, or you wouldn't be a doc. Computing is well within your grasp. Proceed patiently, quietly, and steadily, with the help of a nonpunitive guru who'll show you the first steps and stick with you, and you'll eventually be able to make your own personal best use of what's online—and leave the other tricks for people with nothing better to do.

It has not happened yet, but in the near future all physicians will be using networked personal computers regularly in their daily work, and will be routinely accessing all kinds of clinical and research data online. In a few years, the majority of practicing docs will be of the first generation raised on video games; to them, using computers skillfully is as natural as using the phone.

But even if you've decided in any event not to rush to join the computer revolution, and even if you don't follow any other suggestions, at the bare minimum make sure you have someone in your knowledge network who can access MEDLINE for you.

You owe it to your patients.

## Knowledge Isn't Enough—Unless We Change Our Practice

So far, we've been talking about how we can more efficiently acquire new knowledge. Usually we take for granted that if we learn something new and useful, then we will automatically start using it in our practice—won't we?

Well, no, we won't.

For example, you've probably learned several dozen new ways of doing things in your practice from reading this book. How many have you actually tried out?

Research repeatedly demonstrates that we physicians usually make no significant changes in our daily practice, even after obtaining new knowledge from CME.[4(p.501)] We may do better on quizzes, but we don't change the way we handle patients in our offices by using the new knowledge. Knowledge-creators (researchers) and knowledge-transmitters (professors and other teachers) are frustrated and surprised by this annoying fact.

The problem is that in med school and residency we learned certain ways of doing things, and these first impressions got stamped indelibly into our nervous systems. All those techniques were state of the art when we finished training, and we're fond of them.

### The Key

When I first came on staff at a large hospital, they issued me a set of keys for some of the locked areas. Over the years, the locks at that hospital have been changed several times, so I've been issued several new sets of keys.

A few months ago a nursing supervisor noticed one large, old-fashioned key on my key chain. "My goodness, Doctor," she said, "how come you're still carrying that key? It won't open any of the locks. In fact, it hasn't fitted any of the locks for at least ten years!"

I had no answer for that one, except to get rid of the old key I'd been mindlessly carrying around every day for so many years. I've started wondering about how much other outdated and useless stuff—knowledge, habits, beliefs, prejudices—I inadvertently carry around with me in my professional life.

So although they're outmoded now (whether or not we want to admit it), we still hold on to the old ways. Often you'll hear, "I don't need to be using that yet—it's not really proven," or "I practice conservatively—I pride myself on never being the first to apply a new technique." This kind of stance makes less sense if we recall the story of *H. pylori*—by the time we physicians generally accepted it, this "new" treatment concept was 14 years old! The same lag applies to giving up old treatments such as eye patches after corneal abrasions, spinal fusion for low back pain, etc.

A prank we sometimes play on ourselves: We try out something brand new, and if it fizzles on the first go-around, tell ourselves and anyone else who'll listen, "Oh, I tried that new procedure (drug, instrument, treatment); it's no good. I'm sticking to the good old tried-and-true, etc." Or if another doc in our medical community has jumped ahead of us and started using the new method, the NIH (Not Invented Here) syndrome may make us sniff: "Oh, she uses everything that comes down the pike; I get better results using the older, simpler ways."

Does any of this ring a bell? It won't hurt to **analyze your own practice regularly and decide if you're needlessly hanging on to some outdated clinical techniques**. Again, this is something you'll mostly have to do for yourself—no one else can look over your shoulder and make the call. But if you want to find out quickly whether you're using outdated knowledge, hang out with a sharp senior resident (or fellow, or other newly-minted doc) in your field for a while; their knowledge base is current, and if you're receptive, you'll pick up a lot of new ideas and start using them. (Of course, after they've been out there a few years, their stuff will also be out of date, and they will in turn have to seek out even younger practitioners to keep up with the latest stuff.)

The trick is to know when what you learned as state of the art has truly become a medical Studebaker.[5] It's also a matter of knowing exactly which tiny portion of all the vast ocean of new knowledge is going to be of practical use in treating a specific patient.

But that's a question of wisdom.

---

**Notes**

1. "Docs Are Finally Finding the Internet," *Medical Meetings* 24, no. 8 (1997): 21.
2. A.R. Barrie and A.M. Ward, "Questioning Behavior in General Practice," *British Medical Journal* 315, no. 6 (1997): 1,512–1,515.
3. P.J. Goodnick et al., "Treatment of Depression in Patients with Diabetes Mellitus," *Journal of Clinical Psychiatry* 56, no. 4 (1995): 128–136.
4. E. Evans et al., "Does a Mailed Continuing Education Program Improve Physician Performance?" *Journal of the American Medical Association* 255, no. 4 (1986): 501–504.
5. F. Mullan, "The Journey Back," *Journal of the American Medical Association* 278, no. 4 (1997): 281–283.

## ✦ 11 ✦

# Beyond Knowledge: Clinical Wisdom and Intuition

A generalist asks for a consult on a patient with a puzzling clinical picture of weakness and confusion. The internist consultant works the patient up for hyperparathyroidism, even though two screening chem panels show normal serum calciums. The internist turns out to be correct in his diagnosis. When asked how he made the call in spite of normal serum calciums, he says, "I've seen one or two cases like this before."

A pediatrician examines a little girl with low-grade fever and an apparent URI. The lungs are clear on exam but—on a hunch—he gets a chest film. The x-ray shows a LLL pneumonia, which becomes clinically apparent only the next day. When asked how he decided to get a chest film in this particular case, he shrugs and says, "I don't know—just something about the patient, I guess."

### Experience Gives Us Something Extra

You've heard about or seen cases like these, perhaps even in your own practice. No course, lecture, textbook, or research paper can teach the kind of clinical judgment demonstrated by these two seasoned practitioners.

While you could argue that they were just very observant—or very lucky—most practitioners would agree that, occasionally, we all make sharp clinical decisions that don't seem to be based on didactic knowledge. Beyond the talents, skills, education, and training that we all bring to our daily work, some physicians seem to have developed their clinical judgment to such a point that they can only be described as possessing something extra: clinical wisdom.

> Experience is a hard teacher: She gives the test first, and the lesson afterwards.

But docs tend to be modest—even about other doctors. Rarely will we say, "She's a very wise physician," but we may say instead, "She's the best there is at handling that kind of patient," or "There's one person who'll know how to straighten out a case that's this messed up—let's call her."

You probably know two or three physicians who seem to work at this high level of expertise much of the time—in fact, when we get sick, these are the physicians we personally consult. But probably we've never asked ourselves these questions: Is there really such a thing as clinical wisdom? If so, what does it consist of? Can we develop more of it ourselves? And if we can, how do we go about it?

### Evidence and Experience

The new discipline of evidence-based medicine (EBM) de-emphasizes clinical experience, wisdom, and intuition, insisting that we make our decisions by consulting clinical research databases. "Unsystematic clinical experience" is not sufficient for clinical decision making, according to EBM.[1(p.2,420)]

But clinical experience can be crucial to outcomes. Just ask an advocate of EBM this question: "Who would you rather have do your angioplasty—a cardiologist with excellent training (and also a superior grasp of the clinical research) who does 30 angioplasties a year? Or one with the same training but who does 280 procedures a year?" Forget the research; they'll opt for the cardiologist with more ("unsystematic") experience.

Our EBM person knows (because the literature itself indicates) that he has a significantly better chance of surviving the procedure by going with experience. (In fact, the rate of major complications is more than 300% higher for less experienced cardiologists.[2]) This holds true outside of cardiology, also—among HIV patients, for instance, those with more experienced practitioners have significantly better survival rates.[3] Experience has given these physicians something extra.

We don't have to be in practice very long to discover that while good research is about isolating one independent variable and controlling it, a real patient has variables all over the place, and they're never fully controlled. It fact, it takes clinical experience just to know how and when and whether to apply research findings to an actual patient.

## Why Is This Patient Drowsy?

An internist friend was making rounds with some residents recently when they found an elderly woman sleeping in her bed. She was difficult to rouse. Was the patient overdosed on meds, had she just had a stroke, was this a normal finding for someone this age...what was their opinion?

One resident confidently quoted the literature: "Drug overdose is statistically the most likely reason for her drowsiness, so we should review her meds."

Another disagreed: "Actually, the literature points to the likelihood of a small stroke or TIA here. We need a consult to rule out a neurologic basis for her drowsiness."

"OK," said my internist friend, "granted that the books tell you that meds and TIAs can cause abnormal drowsiness—but is this patient abnormally drowsy? Or is this how someone her age snoozes at this time of day? What exactly do the books mean, anyway, when they say 'drowsy'?"

The residents mumbled something about ventilation rates and ancillary signs, but actually they were stumped by the practical question—and were probably hoping they'd get paged out of rounds real soon.

Just then the "drowsy" patient awoke and started cursing the residents in loud, clear tones for disturbing her daily nap.

Information is what someone has seen, and knowledge is what someone has seen and then thought about; both information and knowledge have short shelf-lives these days. However, if we use clinical knowledge over time, and continue to process that experience, it distills down into something at once more practical and more subtle, which lasts a lot longer, and may even be of permanent value: Call it wisdom.

We often work at a level where we need more than practice guidelines and research databases to help our patient, and we have no choice but to rely on our own (and our knowledge network's) experience, judgment, and wisdom.

### So What Exactly Is Clinical Wisdom—And How Do I Get It?

Clinical wisdom seems to be like charisma in a movie star or virtuosity in a pianist: We may not know exactly what it is, but we recognize that some people definitely have it—and they must have gotten it somewhere. But can we also become wise clinicians?

My best answer: Why not?

Physicians who are considered wise trained in the same schools and residencies we did, read the same books, and have five fingers on each hand, just like you and me. Clearly, though, they're doing something extra. In discussions with physicians, these possible means of increasing our clinical wisdom were mentioned:

1. **Actively seek more clinical experience.** If you're a surgeon, you probably remember that during your residency you'd cruise the wards late at night hoping for a juicy procedure or two before everyone else got back the next morning. Later in our careers, we sometimes start avoiding difficult cases or procedures. But volume makes for skill, and practice makes perfect (almost).

2. **Process your experience (think deeply about it, talk about it, record it).** Wisdom has been defined as distilled experience—but to distill something useful out of raw clinical experience, we'll need to take the time to think more deeply about our cases.

> ❝Knowledge comes, but wisdom lingers.❞
>
> Tennyson, "Locksley Hall"

How about checking your Needs card before starting on that exercise walk or drive home, and spending the solitary time thinking about how you handled a recent case? One dermatologist mentioned to me that he keeps on his desk a file of write-ups and photos of his most puzzling cases and pulls them out now and then to mull over. A Chinese proverb says, "Revisiting old information yields new knowledge."

Beyond knowing the rules, we need to think about and clarify the exceptions. As the old clinical chestnut has it, "Nothing is never always." Beyond diagnosis, we need to think more about prognosis and the finer grain of the natural histories of illnesses as they appear in actual individual patients. But these areas of clinical expertise are famously hard to access in the literature, even by computer; thinking and discussing (thinking out loud with someone else) work better.

## Poor Prognosis

A surgeon told an elderly patient that the laser procedure he was about to perform was "the next best thing to magic," and that the patient would feel great relief. Unfortunately, the procedure, although technically excellent, did not improve his symptoms, and the elderly man became severely depressed.

Thinking is a marvelous habit which—if we actually do it—can make us vastly more productive physicians than many of our colleagues. A woman of my acquaintance recently underwent several days (and a couple of thousand dollars' worth) of negative procedures before the specialist finally took the time to sit down with her and get a history and think about the facts of her case— which clearly indicated she needed to see a different specialist altogether.

Acting before thinking is inefficient medicine, though it may have been a profitable way to proceed in a fee-for-service environment. Now that specialists are being capitated and case-rated, more thought and fewer procedures actually mean higher reimbursements. They have always meant higher quality.

3. **Closely study your (and others') mistakes.** Nobody enjoys making mistakes. We don't much like talking about them, either.

Like airline pilots and nuclear plant operators, doctors are not expected to make errors, and our patients don't want to hear about them, especially at certain times, and for excellent psychological reasons ("Ms. Brown, let me introduce your surgeon; he's quite good, though he has made one or two huge errors in the OR—Ms. Brown, *come back here!*").

> **"**Knowledge grows more by the recognition of errors than by the accumulation of facts.**"**
>
> David Short[4(p.250)]

But all doctors make errors, and the habit of going deeply into any cases where errors have been made is gold. Experience gives you good judgment, but bad judgments give you experience.

4. **Go deep, go broad.** One message of this book has been that just a little bit of your time, invested in thinking about and analyzing whatever you're doing, can yield dividends in making you more efficient, more focused, and happier. Thinking deep and long is such hard work that we usually avoid it. But reflecting about our cases isn't a luxury; it will make us more accurate and more effective practitioners.

Further, because medicine is about humans, we need to broaden our personal knowledge base about the human race. How long has it been since you read a novel so insightful it made you weep?

Do you think deeply, from time to time, about your own personal philosophy, your principles, and how (and whether) they fit with your patients' values and needs? Successful practice requires more than just quoting statistical evidence; you must be able to adapt the evidence to your patient's individuality.

### Something We Never Do

When I was in medical school, a visiting Japanese research fellow asked about my plans. I told him, "Well, I'll finish med school, then residency, then start a practice."

"But won't you take any time off?" he asked incredulously.

I had no idea what he was talking about. "What do you mean, take time off? Why should I take time off?"

"To think about what you are doing."

If we rush headlong through our careers without ever examining the bigger picture, we risk becoming mere machine tenders—or even machines.

5. **Hang out with the wise docs—and also the young ones.** I'm a believer in intercerebral osmosis. The most expert professionals ask different questions, see things from new angles, suggest things we would never have thought of, and make decisions differently. Kirpal Singh often said, "This can't be taught—but it can be caught."[5] Find 'em and hang with 'em—maybe you'll catch it.

> Instead of envying your more productive colleagues,
> try emulating them.

Another advantage of hanging around with the best docs you can find is that you'll begin to soak up a bit of their aura. Not only will you find yourself unconsciously imitating some of their methods and habits, but other people will begin to associate you with your high-functioning friends, so your own reputation will be shinier.

Osler advised all older practitioners to spend time "with the boys" [6(p.144)]—by which he meant doctors between 25 and 40 (now we would say "with the boys and young women"). They're freshly and thoroughly trained in all the new stuff, are not clinging onto any old stuff, and their enthusiasm will rub off on you and get you moving. Seek them out.

6. **Attend, supervise, teach, lecture.** Having any size audience for your clinical knowledge automatically motivates you to sharpen and systematize your thinking. If you've ever tried to sum up for a young resident many years of your own clinical work, then you've started polishing your rough-cut experience into gems of wisdom. Having these at your command will make you more productive in your daily clinical work.

If you're nervous about being an attending, sign up for just a month. You can bone up quickly a day or two before starting, if you're rusty, and there's even a book you can read on how to be a good attending.[7] Your experience will be valued by your students and residents, and you'll be learning as much as you'll be teaching—so everyone will benefit.

7. **Learn to manage uncertainty.** "Judgment is difficult," Hippocrates reminds us across the ages. Often, in the pressurized atmosphere of a particularly risky case, we just don't know enough to act; yet we're penalized if we don't act, so we may prematurely jump to diagnose or treat. Part of clinical wisdom is knowing how to manage (and control for) our own uncertainty, acting neither too soon nor too late.

If we pay attention to our really hairy cases, we can learn something from them about our own patterns of reacting to clinical uncertainty. As the high-wire artist said before he hit the ground, timing is everything. Do we sometimes hang on too long, paralyzed? Or do we tend to let go of the trapeze before we know enough about where we'll land? Are we dogmatic, not open to others' suggestions?

8. **Analyze your own practice style (reflect, cogitate, meditate).** Self-analysis can be more potent than Freud ever dreamed, which is why the 3,000-year-old inscription over the Delphic Oracle reads, "Man, know yourself." Some things to try:

✦ You can use your Needs card to spot areas of deficiency in your clinical knowledge base as you become aware of them in practice.

✦ You might also think realistically about your limitations as a physician and as a person so you can steer away from cases you can't handle—but not hand off the ones you can do competently.

✦ If you're older, you've naturally had more experience than younger docs—and this includes more bad experiences, too. As a result, you may have become too tentative and conservative in your approach to some clinical problems; look for this tendency, and correct for it.

It would seem logical that most of us could profit from learning more about how we do our work, and identifying our own practice patterns. (The exceptions: those very able physicians who work fast, on "automatic pilot"—they might trip over their own feet if they slowed down to analyze their work methods.) Yet there is no hard evidence that physicians can actually use this kind of self-knowledge to change their practice patterns (e.g., their problem-solving approach) for the better. My suspicion is that this kind of change is a long, slow process, and therefore not amenable to research—but that the well-examined professional life is a step toward clinical wisdom.

9. **Read, study, train—all the time.** We all would like to have muscles like Arnold Schwarzenegger's, but are we willing to work out every day—even on vacations—like he does?

Recall for a moment how hard you worked to get the knowledge you got in med school and residency. Have you kept up your level of effort in this area of your professional life? If you're getting in ten hours a month of education and training (the average for all U.S. physicians), could you double it? That would still be only five hours a week, less than one tenth of your working time. You can squeeze it in if you manage your time better, eliminating activities that are less productive.

## Clinical Intuition

You're working along on a difficult and complex case, but something in the back of your brain keeps telling you that you're on the wrong track. You carefully review your information and your line of thinking, and logically it all seems to add up. Yet in the end it turns out you actually were on the wrong track—and your clinical intuition was correct.

If clinical wisdom is a controversial subject, then clinical intuition is a scandal.

We all know about it, but we're not supposed to talk about it, because it sounds mystical and supernatural, like making prophecies or reading auras or tea leaves. Actually, clinical intuition has nothing to do with all the so-called "intuitive arts" or other such bunkum.

Forgive me if I speak just once as a psychiatrist to remind everyone that not all of what's going on in our minds is necessarily directly available to our consciousness. We're quite capable of observing, reacting, and processing without being aware that we're doing so. In the simplest case, everyone has had the experience of suddenly—and seemingly out of nowhere—remembering that they have to call the lab or check on a patient, just at the precise moment when the task needs to be done. It's as if you had set a silent alarm in your unconscious.

Reputable research is now suggesting that intuition does exist. Called "nondeclarative dispositional knowledge," it seems to be centered in the ventromedial frontal cortex and works parallel to—but faster than—overt reasoning processes to "bias the circuits that support conscious cognition."[8(p.1,293)]

In other words, intuition.

The French, of course, have always had a word for it: *flair clinique.*

Whatever we call it, there seems to be a little voice in the back of our head that talks to us sometimes. It's probably nothing more mysterious than our clinical faculties working just outside of normal consciousness.

One of the great discoveries in psychology post-Freud has been that we can exercise some influence (e.g., by repetitive verbal inputs) over the less conscious parts of our mind. So you can intentionally try to strengthen that helpful little voice. The next time it says to you, "Go back to the ward and check Ms. Green's belly"— go back. If it's a very strong hunch—go back. If you review your clinical thinking, and a re-exam is not unreasonable—go back.

If you find Ms. Green's belly is negative, nothing has been lost but a minute or two; if you do find something significant in her belly, you'll be more likely to pay attention in the future.

Certain mental practices, such as silent meditation, also may enhance this faculty. When you sit in meditation, clear your head, and quiet down the constant 30-thoughts-per-minute vocalizing of your conscious mind, it's possible to get in touch with more deeply coded information. Since this type of knowing sometimes presents as a "feeling," being in better touch with your feelings— and freely talking about them—could also help.

So what will happen if you **listen to the little voice in the back of your head**?

Next time, it will be louder.

> **Warning and Disclaimer:** *The foregoing is for informa-tion only. Please do not infer that any practitioner can or should rely preferentially on limited personal experience, hunches, instinct, or intuition when sound clinical re-search exists to guide their decision making. Never gamble with your patients' health.*

## Mentors and Protégés

If you were going on vacation in the Greek Isles, you'd want brochures and guidebooks to read up on that area, or you'd watch a travelogue, or search the Web for some informative sites with recent news about routes, shopping, weather, etc.

But if you met someone who actually lived in the Greek Isles, and who offered to go there with you, introduce you to the locals, be your on-call guide and sponsor, all free of charge—wouldn't that be the best of all?

That's what a mentor is.

In the business world, it's common practice for a more experi-enced executive to take on a promising younger person and act as their guide or mentor. This is different from attending or supervis-ing a resident; the mentor is usually not concerned with training or evaluating the up-and-coming protégé.

What the mentor offers is more personal: She welcomes the younger person into the work, guides and encourages her in a way that maximizes individual potential, inspires her, gives her real psychological support when she needs it, sets an example, champions the younger person's cause—"facilitates the Dream," in seminar-speak. A mentor is a sort of aunt/uncle-role model-adviser-guru-ally. In the sometimes forbidding, disinterested world of medicine, a mentor is an island of human warmth and a psychological anchor.

I've had three mentors in my professional life. The first gave me a job doing clinical research when I came back from military service. He welcomed me socially to our profession and to a new city, showed me how to start my practice, sent me my first private patients, and even helped me choose some decent civilian clothes.

Fifteen years later, when I became chief of staff, our medical director took me under his wing and let me in on some secrets of how to get things done on the administrative side of medicine.

My mentor these days helps me with (among other things) ethical questions in my practice, investments and retirement planning, and computers (I'm writing this book on a computer he gave me and tutored me on). Interestingly, although he mentors me, he's younger than I am.

## How Do You Get a Mentor or a Protégé?

If you're a seasoned person in your field, out of the many younger practitioners whom you meet, one or two will probably seek you out for advice. If you encourage this, you'll soon have a protégé. Looking for a mentor? Start with your personal panel of experts. If you go to a senior person for advice, he probably won't say, "I'm mentoring you" in so many words, but as the two of you meet together and become friends, and as you ask for guidance on difficult decisions, the association will gradually become a mentor-protégé relationship.

A colleague wrote: "I see two former residents in a loose mentoring relationship, and we talk mostly about finances, career decisions, family matters. They enjoy talking about their blossoming professional lives. Both of them are recent immigrants to the U.S., so I go out of my way to make them feel welcome to this country.

When I'm with them I feel young myself. I get much personal joy working with them." Sounds like a win-win.

Even if you think you're too old, consider taking on a mentor—maybe in computers, or some newer aspects of your field. In fact, whatever your age, **consider taking on a mentor or a protégé**. There's so much more to doctoring—and to living—than what's in books, lectures, and seminars. If you're wiser, you should be passing your wisdom on. If you're less experienced, you can save yourself a lot of time and uncertainty by having the input of a seasoned practitioner who's already been there, done that, got the T-shirt.

Nurses have told me that younger docs often have a great feel for the latest technical knowledge, but can learn a lot about relationships. Conversely, older docs often have developed "the touch" in relationships with patients and co-workers—but may need to learn more about the latest wrinkles in diagnosis and treatment. So it makes sense for docs to pair off into mentor–protégé relationships, which invariably are two-way streets. The young, eager residents whom I presume to tutor in the finer points of the clinical art have more than once lit a fire under my rear end, and gotten me to try some of the newest treatments available in our field.

As a by-product of mentoring a less experienced colleague, physicians report that they themselves grow; they get more empathy, more feeling for the life cycle within our profession. Raising children can make a person more mature, and mentoring can make us wiser physicians.

### Friends

Last spring at a productivity seminar in Oregon, the audience was loud, enthusiastic, and mostly young. But one practitioner had brought an older man, who looked to be in his late 80s. The younger doc had to lean over and repeat everything into his companion's ear during the seminar, and I could tell they were good friends.

Afterward I asked the younger man to introduce me. "This is my longtime mentor, Dr. D. He's been retired for some time now, but whenever I come into Portland, I pick him up and we spend the whole day together."

The older physician did not speak, but his glistening eyes told me how much this collegial friendship meant to him in his sunset years.

## Find Your Own Personal Best Learning Methods

*Because of the explosion in knowledge and the accelerating velocity of its dissemination, we physicians can no longer keep up with new information in our field by using the same techniques of learning that we've been using up to now.*

That sentence is so important, please go back and read it again, so the idea really sinks into your brain.

The familiar, comfortable ways we now have of acquiring and updating our knowledge and skills will not work in the future. To keep up with modern medicine and to become more productive, we need to **develop more efficient ways of learning**.

This area will probably be one of the growth industries of the future. It already has a name: "metacognition," or learning about how we learn, and feeding back that information to make us more efficient learners.[9]

This is a new concept for most of us. In med school and residency no one ever asked you whether you preferred to learn by lecture, reading, group discussion, or hands-on demo; you pretty much just had to learn the stuff any way it was being taught—or else.

---

❝Knowledge, it is predicted, will shortly double every year. ...Clearly, we must develop new strategies for dealing with the sheer volume of data, concepts, principles, and skills that health care providers need to have at their command.❞

Christine H. McGuire, MD[10(pp.9–10)]

---

Since your brain is a little bit different from mine, it makes sense that you may have a different optimal way of learning—but whether each person actually has her own individual all-time most efficient learning channels is a somewhat more controversial area than some authors of quick-learning systems would have us believe.

Also, there seem to be so many different learning styles, it can get confusing. If you prefer to learn things step by step, you're supposed to be a left-brain learner, whereas if you like to see the big picture or the end result first and work toward it, you're more right-brain. If you prefer reading and writing things down to hearing and discussing, you're more visual than auditory, and vice versa. If you don't enjoy left-brain audio or written presentations, but prefer actually getting your hands on things and touching them while you learn, you're more right-brain tactile. Some people seem to learn more quickly from clinical vignettes, while others prefer diagrams and algorithms, or aphorisms or mnemonics, or watching a master clinician at work, etc.

Usually about a third of the physicians who come to productivity seminars ask for a written syllabus which they can follow and write notes on, while another third want to hear anecdotes and seem not to want to distract themselves writing. Roughly another third will come up afterward to discuss the seminar and ask questions. This suggests to me that we physicians do tend to have somewhat individualized personal learning styles.

But do you know which methods of learning are most efficient for you? **Look at what you're doing now to acquire and update your clinical skills, and think about what actually works best for you.** Reading? Listening? Taking notes? Taking tests? Hands-on? Mentoring? Discussing a case with another practitioner? Going online? CD-ROMs? Simulations? Have you tried all of these methods? Combinations of them?

It's been pretty much taken for granted that everyone can learn any new clinical information equally fast whether they're staring at a computer screen, or reading and annotating a printed text, or discussing cases with a colleague, or listening to a lecture. People trying to sell you expensive CD-ROM learning programs will assure you that their medium is an efficient way for every practitioner to get new clinical knowledge.

Baloney. We're all different. Therefore, you can make your learning more efficient by finding out what actually works best for your learning style.

 **Exercise 11–1** Analyze your CME activities to detect those that seem to yield the fastest, easiest, and most definite increase in your personal knowledge base. After you attend a lecture or workshop, read a journal article, or search an electronic database, be conscious of how much useful new information you actually get for the time and effort involved in each activity—and *whether the new information changes the way you practice.* When you do find yourself using new knowledge in your practice, stop to recall how you learned it.

Then try to expose yourself intentionally to more of the type of learning experience that you find most efficient (e.g., if you learn well in discussions, sign up for

more group teaching situations at your next association meeting, etc.).

## Keep Moving and Enjoy

Research shows that no single learning intervention is as effective in changing physicians' behavior as multiple interventions.[11]
Also, one law of mental function is that we get bored with any one
thing done repeatedly, so you will need to **change your methods of learning** from time to time.

Another strong finding coming out of research into physician
learning: It helps if we can **enjoy the learning experience**.
Learning is hard and sometimes frustrating work, but a skilled and
inspiring teacher, a jovial and supportive colleague, and a learning method that suits us can all make knowledge acquisition
more fun.

Come to think of it, a few palm trees probably don't hurt, either.

 **Exercise 11–2** Circle the suggestions below that you
will try in your own practice. Add your own suggestions at the end of the list. Keep this book in your office
and refer back to this list when you have a moment.
Analyze which suggestions are working best for you,
and consider whether some others on this list may be
worth trying.

1. Analyze your CME activities to ensure that they
   are maximally useful in your practice.
2. Seek and use educational materials that fit your
   unique needs.
3. Hook up educational activities directly to your
   caseload.
4. Keep a Needs card with you.
5. Skip 50% of papers in most journals.
6. Throw out half your journals.

7. Don't try to read articles from beginning to end.
8. Surf, skim, scan, skip, speed-read.
9. Use your Needs card as a guide while scanning.
10. Put together a personal knowledge network.
11. Pick the best articles that impact on the needs of your practice, and rip them out.
12. File them in two folders, and keep the folders on your desk.
13. When you see a case, pull the relevant articles and study your materials carefully.
14. Think about what you're reading.
15. Consciously get rid of outdated ideas and techniques.
16. Get rid of articles in your files over four years old.
17. Give input to your CME committee.
18. Send them a summary of your Needs card.
19. Tell them about good speakers and articles.
20. Make sure speakers are briefed.
21. Get maximum exposure to an excellent teacher-speaker.
22. Attend meetings of organizations that customize CME to your needs.
23. Set up a personal panel of experts.
24. Maximize your expertise in your field.
25. Cultivate your knowledge network.
26. Sit on peer review, and take your Needs card to meetings.
27. Analyze your near misses.
28. Discuss errors with another practitioner.
29. Find one colleague-friend with whom you regularly discuss your cases in depth.
30. Take written quizzes and mock boards.
31. Own and study the most recent general handbook in your field.

32. Give a lecture.
33. Do research.
34. Commit yourself to learn a new procedure.
35. Find a skilled practitioner to imitate.
36. Have sessions in private.
37. Analyze sequential steps.
38. Practice sub-units.
39. Practice the whole procedure over and over.
40. Use a new skill soon and often.
41. Be prepared for suboptimal outcomes at first.
42. Be prepared to work hard.
43. Use MEDLINE in your daily clinical work.
44. Analyze your clinical practice for outdated techniques.
45. Actively seek more clinical experience.
46. Think deeply about your experience.
47. Associate with wise colleagues.
48. Attend, supervise, teach, lecture.
49. Learn to manage uncertainty.
50. Analyze your own clinical style.
51. Read, study, train more.
52. Don't ignore your intuition.
53. Take on a mentor or a protégé.
54. Identify and use your personal best learning methods.
55. Change your learning methods occasionally for multiple impact and variety
56. Enjoy the learning process.

(add your own ideas here)

_____

_____

_____

**Notes**

1. Evidence-Based Medicine Working Group, "Evidence-Based Medicine," *Journal of the American Medical Association* 268, no. 17 (1992): 2,420–2,425.

2. R. Voelker, "Practice Makes Perfect," *Journal of the American Medical Association* 277, no. 24 (1997): 1,926.

3. J. Stephenson, "Survival of Patients with AIDS Depends on Physicians' Experience Treating the Disease," *Journal of the American Medical Association* 275, no. 10 (1996): 745–746.

4. D. Short, "Learning from Our Mistakes," *British Journal of Hospital Medicine,* 51, no. 5 (1994): 250.

5. K. Singh, *The Teachings of Kirpal Singh, Volume III: The New Life* (Bowling Green, VA: Sawan Kirpal Publications, 1981), 151.

6. W. Osler, *Aequanimitas* (Philadelphia, PA: Blakiston, 1932), 144.

7. L. Osborn and N. Whitman, *Ward Attending* (Salt Lake City, UT: University of Utah School of Medicine, 1991).

8. A. Bechara et al., "Deciding Advantageously Before Knowing the Advantageous Strategy," *Science* 275 (1997): 1,293–1,295.

9. D. Irby, "Ideas for Medical Education," *Academic Medicine* 72, no. 1 (1997): 30–35.

10. Anonymous, "Research in Medical Education," *Academic Medicine* 71, supplement (1996): 9–10.

11. J.A.M. Gray, "Continuing Education: What Techniques Are Effective?" *Lancet,* 23 August, 1980, 447–448.

# Part 4

# Relationship Management for Physicians

# ✦ 12 ✦

# The Hidden Secret of Physician Productivity

No matter how many hours of time you put in, no matter how highly skilled and knowledgeable you are, no matter how hard you work—if your patients and your staff don't care for you, then you won't be a maximally productive physician.

Conversely, if you are well liked and admired by your patients and co-workers, and if you reciprocate in kind, daily practice becomes a joy; such a practice will motivate and enable you to be much more productive without any sense of increased effort on your part. So, while the discipline of medicine may be an applied biological science, practicing productively turns out to be a matter of managing your professional relationships, and has more to do with applied psychology than with biology.

## Medicine = Relationships

We physicians are people who like working with people. Early in our careers we purposely passed up the opportunity to spend our days working alone in an ivory laboratory or at a computer console, and chose instead to enter the hurly-burly of a people profession. In medical school, watching master clinicians work skillfully with people in pain or panic, we learned patience and understanding.

But then, during our training, we picked up a lot of lousy interpersonal habits. If we wanted to be considered "efficient" residents, we had to reduce the attention we gave each patient to the bare minimum necessary for getting our work done. We may have learned to be arrogant and abusive to nurses and other co-workers (later we'll see how). And we picked up some unwarranted prejudices toward many of our colleagues. We need to keep in mind that residencies and fellowships make us technical experts, but learning the art of building and maintaining a practice starts in earnest only after our formal training is finished.

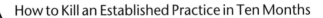 How to Kill an Established Practice in Ten Months

Last Christmas my friend Beth called from Florida, where for 15 years she has been managing a busy one-man office for a GYN surgeon. On the machine she sounded stressed, so I called her right back. Here's the story Beth told me:

In June her previous doc, an older man, had sold his flourishing practice to a woman who was just finishing her fellowship in GYN surgery, and Beth stayed with the practice. The young surgeon was quite good at procedures and was also teaching and doing research in the field—but unfortunately, Beth said, she had no concept of how to handle patients. She was curt, standoffish, insensitive, and preferred to discuss delicate questions over the phone, or not at all. Her style was in sharp contrast to the older surgeon, who had put a lot of effort into building trust in his patients, many of whom were worried and upset over their condition and needed sensitive handling.

There were scenes with the new doc, and patients began picking up their records and leaving; in a few months the practice basically fell apart. New referrals dried up as ex-patients complained to other physicians, and where there had been ten new patients a week, there were soon only three. Beth tried to talk to the doc, and even had other surgeons in the community talk to her, but the young woman would not listen. She seemed oblivious to the reasons for what was happening—and in fact put most of her attention into her teaching and research.

Shortly after the New Year, Beth accepted an offer to work for another surgeon in the community. Soon afterward her old office closed. The young woman GYN surgeon returned to a full-time academic position. The practice, which two previous surgeons had built up for almost 40 years, lasted only ten months with the new surgeon.

Professional relationships are that important.

If you look again at the Physician Productivity Equation in Chapter 2, you'll see that our time and knowledge get delivered and amplified (or diverted and diluted) through these relationships. The people you work with can save you a lot of time and effort, or they can cost you a lot of extra work; and they can make your workplace a pleasant haven or a little bit of hell right here on earth.

Recall for a moment the last time you had a major falling-out with someone at work, and how the whole place got so poisoned with tension that you and everyone else hated even to be there. In such an atmosphere, with so much energy tied up in negativity, it's painful or impossible to be productive. In contrast, when you have excellent relationships with your patients and colleagues and are working with a great clinical team, work becomes a joy.

I continue to be surprised by how little formal training we receive during med school and residency in how to optimize our professional interactions with patients, co-workers, and colleagues. I've enjoyed speaking and writing about this third tool of physician productivity the most, because it's so generally ignored—and because I believe that we can all (myself included) use a lot of help in this neglected area.

Not only do bad relationships slow us down and make everyone's work much harder, I've come to the conclusion that they are the ultimate source of our inefficiency. Friction with our patients and staff generates discomfort, stress, errors, misunderstandings, and lawsuits. Aloofness from our colleagues cuts down our potential pool of knowledge and help, and weakens our profession.

This book is primarily about productivity, but there's more to our professional lives than efficiency; we also have hearts, and so I must add that good professional relationships give us—beyond any gains in productivity—pleasures and satisfactions that are valuable for their own sake. These values never appear in a clinical record, a research report, or on the bottom line, but they are nonetheless real; you can *feel* them.

### How Do You Solve an Invisible Problem?

You know most of this already, and you're weary of hearing it; every recent book and journal article seems to be telling us docs that we have to improve our relationships—unfortunately, they don't really tell us how to go about it, so they're not much help.

One thing is sure: Just saying to yourself, "Today, I'm going to start getting along really well with everyone" won't work, because we rarely know much about our own problems in professional relationships, nor what they're doing to our potential productivity. Like the young woman surgeon in the story, we can be oblivious to major problems that others feel very acutely.

While we know that we have too little time and that there's too much available knowledge, in general we're not aware of our professional relationships—period. The whole drama seems to be happening below our radar. In fact, in a recent survey of young physicians, relationships came a distant last on their list of problems at work.[2] Being ignorant of our difficulties could explain why we have so many interpersonal problems in the first place, and why our public image, both as individuals and as a profession, has gotten raggedy.

### What Our Office Managers Think about Us

A few months ago I gave a seminar to a large group of physicians' office managers. When we got to the section on relationships, I asked for volunteers to yell out some characteristics of the typical physician's personality, so I could make a list on the flip chart. I naively assumed I would hear the usual traits we associate with our profession: intelligent, dedicated, caring, thorough, etc. But these managers had different ideas.

"ARROGANT!" yelled several.

"GREEDY!" shouted another.

"Stubborn!" muttered another.

"Angry!"

"Controlling!"

"Rude!" and on and on.

They continued shouting out negative characteristics, one after another, until the flip chart page was completely full, and I had to stop writing.

> Frankly embarrassed by what these people—who work every day with physicians—thought of us, I said, "OK, that's enough negative characteristics. Now how about some positive physician traits....Anyone? ...Anyone at all?"
>
> There were 175 people in the room, but the silence was pin-drop. After a few moments it became embarrassing.
>
> Finally one office manager raised her hand. "Well, I'm not sure, but in some situations...I think...the doctor ...acts as the patient's advocate."
>
> This was the single positive comment about us that large crowd of people who work with us could come up with.

We're often the last to know about our relationship problems, partly because our white coat or scrubs deflect a certain amount of face-to-face criticism, and partly because we tend to be more intent on getting our important work done than on noticing whose feelings may get bruised in our headlong rush. Also, our co-workers (especially nurses) usually are resigned to putting up with our annoying behavior. I know of one hospital that keeps a secret list of its staff physicians' peculiarities and idiosyncrasies available in every nursing station, so nurses can work around the doctors' problems.

But just because they won't say it to our faces doesn't mean our co-workers don't express their opinions of physicians in other ways. If you could be a fly on the wall after you leave your workplace, you would hear quite a bit of gossip, complaints, and general backbiting about physicians. As the Scottish poet Robert Burns wrote of the fine lady with the louse on her bonnet, "O wad some Pow'r the giftie gie us/To see oursels as others see us."

Docs are genuinely surprised to find out what some of our co-workers actually think of us, but it's worth trying to find out. As long as we stay oblivious to the problems we're having in our work relationships, they'll keep interfering with our efficiency—because good work relationships are not just more pleasant, they're also more efficient. Research shows that good relationships produce better clinical outcomes, even more reliably than technical support.[3]

So how can we make sure we have good professional relationships?

## People Are Never Tools

You've noticed that in the chapters on time management and knowledge management, I've already slipped in a lot about professional relationships: personal knowledge networks, peer friendships, communicating with nurses, phone etiquette, etc. But these five chapters won't be about "managing" relationships in the same sense that we have aggressively taken command of our own time and our personal knowledge base. This is going to be a different kind of undertaking because (as you've noticed) people are independent, unpredictable, often unfathomable—in short, human. So improving our productivity by improving our professional relationships is not about trying to get everyone else to dance to our tune (which is probably impossible). It's much more a question of understanding how we affect others and then taking control of ourselves so that people work better with us and for us.

A key concept to understand here is that everyone wants above all to be treated humanely; they usually respond with sincere interest, helpfulness, and loyalty to the rare physicians who consistently treat them that way. But while we'd all like to treat all people well all the time, the pressures of our work and our lives, our own personality, or our past experiences with others unfortunately keep us from doing so.

If we want to improve our relationships at work, we'll have to start by understanding the biggest general criticisms of physicians' working style, then analyze our own unique way of working with others, and finally begin weeding out those personal behaviors that are least appealing and least efficient.

## Yeah, But Who Has the Time for Relationships?

"I'm too busy to agonize over how I work with people; I'm a surgeon, not a social worker," one attendee complained to me during a seminar. "And most of the time, I work under a lot of pressure—so I don't really feel like doing that, anyway."

Most of us can relate to this surgeon's plaint: We usually don't have the time or the inclination to put a lot of effort into improving our working relationships. And when we feel frustrated and angry, we're even less likely to want to work calmly and patiently at improving the atmosphere in which we labor.

But a few minutes daily spent on sharpening this third tool can, I guarantee you, save you hours (and finally, years) of inefficient work and low-grade misery. Think about it: Wouldn't you rather have more people working more of the time to get more of your work done for you? Wouldn't that save you time, effort, and unhappiness in the long run—not to speak of making a lot of other people happier, and thereby more productive?

---

In every field of endeavor, friends mean success.

---

So now that you're more efficient at managing your time and acquiring clinically useful knowledge, I would suggest you start investing some of the time and attention you're saving into learning to use your third tool—Relationships—much more skillfully. One caveat: Do not start working on this section when you're rushed, angry, pressured, or trying to kick caffeine. But at the first lull in your clinical work, when you find yourself with a few moments to spare, instead of leafing through your journals, take the time to try a few of these suggestions. I promise the return on your investment will be worth it.

Let's start by looking at how we might improve our relationships with the most important people in our professional lives: our patients.

---

**Notes**

1. C.E. Dwyer, *The Shifting Sources of Power and Influence* (Tampa, FL: American College of Physician Executives, 1991), 9.

2. M. Hojat and J.S. Gonnella, "Gender Comparisons of Young Physicians' Perceptions of Their Medical Education, Professional Life, and Practice," *Academic Medicine* 70, no. 4 (1995): 305–312.

3. W.A. Knaus et al., "An Evaluation of Outcome from Intensive Care in Major Medical Centers," *Annals of Internal Medicine* 104 (1986): 410–418.

# ✦ 13 ✦

# For Patients, Trust Is the Key

Tolstoy said all happy families are pretty much the same. By the same token, all good relationships have the same general characteristics: mutual trust, concern, affection, helpfulness, good communication, etc.

But in the patient–physician relationship, extraordinary trust is the rule.

Think how absolutely trusting a surgical patient must be at the moment he slips under anesthesia and lets his surgeon cut him open from cricoid to crotch, handle his tissues and organs, perhaps stop his heart and reroute his circulation, find and remove the pathology, etc.

Do you have that much trust in anyone?

Non-surgical patients also have to trust our implicit dedication to diagnosing exhaustively and prescribing accurately. In any one case, at any one moment, there's usually room for only one physician to have a full grasp of what's going on and what needs to be done next.

When you're working long and late and alone on a case, you realize that you're the only person in the world who can actually know whether you're making the optimal effort, or if you're funking it. No computer program and no quality assurance committee in the world can see into your mind at that moment to detect the little shortcut, the slight relaxation, the tiny compromise. But you can see it.

> ❝In any situation, it's a physician's job to do what is in the best interest of his patient. Period.❞
>
> James Andrews, MD[1(p.57)]

Patients also trust us to make sure the whole health care system works for them the way it's supposed to—as if we could! But since no one else takes our solemn oath of service to our patient, or is seen as having at least some knowledge of all clinical aspects of health care, patients naturally trust you and me to ensure the highest standards in our office or our hospital, our nursing staff, our drugs, our equipment, etc.

This trust in one's physician is a powerful anodyne, and helps patients talk about distressing things and undergo unpleasant procedures. Trust makes for less fear and psychic pain—and for better compliance and outcomes. Trust is pathognomonic of a good doctor–patient relationship; when your patient says, "I trust you more than I trust Dr. X," that's a major compliment to you.

And trust is more than all these things: Along with specialized knowledge, it's the key to physicians' power to help others. As long as society trusts us, it will keep granting us our privileged autonomy. So if we can inspire and increase our patients' trust, we can restore the waning power of our profession.

All very well, you say—but what exactly do our patients base their trust on?

## How Patients Judge Their Doctors

Which of the following do you think is the single most important criterion by which patients judge you as a physician:

✦ Your technical skill and competence?
✦ Your training?
✦ Your thoroughness?
✦ Your reputation?
✦ Your appearance?

The correct answer: usually, none of the above.

In fact, the single most important criterion by which your patients judge you is...your interviewing skill.

Which makes good sense, if you think about it. As your colleague, I may know a lot about you: where you trained, how consistent and dependable are your skills and judgment, how current your knowledge is, how thorough you are at following through, etc.

> **❝However well physicians have learned the science of medicine, they use themselves to practice the art.❞**
>
> Dennis M. Novack, MD[2(p.502)]

But your patient knows firsthand only what she can learn about you in the few minutes you spend with her, during the clinical interview. She may have picked up some secondhand knowledge from the way your staff talks about you and acts toward you, but essentially, for your patient, the clinical interview *is* the doctor–patient relationship. And during those few minutes, it's not so much what you do as how you do it that they notice. Physicians may be unhappy to hear that their own self-presentation style is the single most important thing to their patients, but that doesn't make it less true.[3]

The tiny window of time with the patient is "make or break" for the physician, yet intensive training in interviewing techniques and self-presentation skills has been absent from most residencies (except psychiatry) until recently; meanwhile, poor interviewing skills are rampant. A study of 29 videotaped office visits showed that not one physician checked to see if their patient understood their instructions, or explained why a follow-up visit was necessary. Half the docs did not tell their patient how long the treatment would last.[4]

Luckily, good interviewing techniques are teachable—we teach them to psych residents every day. If you haven't done it yet, **get training in interviewing skills** in order to optimize your relationships with your patients. It could be the best investment of time and effort you'll make during your career. Not only will you be increasing your own patients' satisfaction, you'll be enhancing the status of our entire profession. And it's not that complicated.

### The Well-Tempered Interview

Workshops in clinical interviewing emphasize that every patient encounter, however brief, has four parts; we should not normally omit any part, even if we're rushing:

1. **Don't skip a brief introduction, with some effort to create or continue the relationship.** As when greeting any other acquaintance, "Nice to meet you" or "I remember you, it's good to see you again" are probably minimal. This isn't just courtesy; it's connecting.
2. **Monitoring the problem** by review of history and new findings, exam, etc. is the "meat" of the traditional clinical interview, but cannot stand alone.
3. Always make some attempt to **inform, educate, and enlist your patient** in the therapeutic effort. ("Here's what we know so far...so I would suggest that you...etc.") We'll see later how crucial this step is to patient retention. In the future, more and more of our practice will consist of educating our patients in how to keep themselves healthier or in

how to become experts at managing their chronic disease. For a young diabetic child and her parents, for instance, only 10% of treatment is medicine—the other 90% is information (how to handle birthday cakes, sleepovers, etc.). And recent studies show that you, the physician, are actually the best person to educate your patient.

4. Always **close the encounter** crisply but kindly. ("So things look pretty good…see you Thursday after the CAT scan is back.") We sometimes try to close a visit by writing a scrip or an order, but this is not necessary if we use our voice and body language skillfully.

Note how much of good clinical interviewing is not about diagnosis and treatment at all, but about managing the relationship between you and your patient. Studies show this technique does not take longer than the brusque, "Just-the-facts-ma'am" biomedical interview, and patients will be much more satisfied with it—and with you.

## Our Patients' Biggest Complaints

"My doctor doesn't listen to me" and "My doctor doesn't spend enough time with me" are consistently our patients' commonest complaints about our clinical style. These two complaints are exacerbated by the speedup in patient visits that almost all physicians have had to deal with in the past five years. Generalists are now down to an average visit of 10 minutes, specialists to 15. (If these are averages, I don't like to think about what the low ends of the curves look like.)

This trend to ultra-fast patient turnover is spreading to other health care professionals: nurse practitioners and physician assistants in large HMOs are also being asked to see many more patients per day.

### 100 Patients per Day

My friend Calvin, a family practitioner, worked for a giant HMO, doing 12-hour shifts in urgent care. His average: six to eight walk-in patients per hour. Sometimes two or three patients were scheduled for each available time slot.

"How do you do that?" I asked him last year. "How do you see almost 100 patients every day?"

"I just start writing the scrip the minute they walk in the door," he confided gloomily. "It's so bad, when I get off work and see people out on the street, I automatically start writing scrips for them, too!"

"How long can you keep this up, Cal?"

"Not long; it's a burnout."

This year, Calvin left the HMO, and now practices overseas.

Another physician told me—only half in jest—that he has started doing his clinic visits sitting in a rolling desk chair. He ro-l-l-l-l-s into an examining room, slows down only long enough to quickly question-examine-and-prescribe, then ro-l-l-l-ls right out the door and into the next examining room! (This would be hilarious, if the implications weren't so tragic.)

A nurse in Nevada told me that when she looks down the corridor of her office suite, it looks like a pinball machine, with her doctors *ping*-ing in and out of examining rooms.

It would be lovely if we could reassure one another that the era of the longer, more leisurely patient visit will return, that this production-line way of practicing is only a temporary glitch in the history of late-20th-century medicine.

But that's not true; shorter visits are here to stay.

Three forces usually dictate changes in our world: technology, economics, and demographics. And all of these change makers are powering historic shifts in the way we practice medicine. Right now, both information- and diagnostic/treatment technologies are speeding us up by several orders of magnitude. Corporatization, competition, and management of medical practice for maximum profit are speeding us up. And population shifts—especially among the elderly and the poor, who need much more medical care—are speeding us up.

These genies are not going back in their bottles. So rather than longing for a vanished era, we need to develop more effective ways of coping with the new realities.

## Making the Shorter Visit Longer

Physicians who see a lot of patients in a short time have talked to us about their best techniques for working within more constrained time schedules. We've questioned patients about their experiences during physician visits. Also, recent research into patient satisfaction with various styles of physician practice indicates that there are ways to make shorter visits more valuable to patients. The following is a synthesis of this information about how you can cope with having to see more patients in less time.

1. **Focus fully on the visit.** Psychologically, it's more difficult to be as effective in a short visit if you're preoccupied with other things. Try to compartmentalize your work; clear up or put aside any distracting clinical concerns, business worries, family emergencies, etc., before starting your office schedule or rounds.

Sometimes you need to get the patient focused, too. If they have ten unrelated complaints, and visit frequently, just say something like, "Which of these problems is disturbing you the most? We can work on that one today."

2. **No interruptions.** Just a reminder that interruptions slow you down, decrease your accuracy and efficiency, and also are resented by patients.

Little details that you may not think of as interruptions upset some patients: for instance, turning your back on them to focus on your computer screen (reposition the console or get a laptop). In fact, patients are starting to complain that because of the electronic-machine tending we now seem to be doing most of the time, doctors and nurses are pretty much ignoring the people we're supposed to be treating. In this way, too much technology can inadvertently lower your productivity.

Some patients will bring their entire extended family into the examining room for support, but if a few aunts and uncles start asking about their own symptoms, the visit turns chaotic. A limit of one supportive family member makes more sense (a healthy one who can translate, if necessary). Have one of your staff primed to talk somewhere else with the others.

3. **Put full attention on your patient. Make eye contact**, however brief.

Imagine this scenario: You're visiting someone you're fond of, whom you've looked forward to seeing. That person spends your entire visit reading a chart, staring at a screen, checking some data, answering a phone, talking to a nurse, writing down information, etc., and never really looks at you. How would you feel at the end of such a visit?

Patients report that if their physician visit goes like this, then it seems too short—no matter how long it actually was!

The problem is that we measure the attention we give to patients quantitatively, in terms of minutes, but they measure it qualitatively. Did my physician pay any real attention to me? Did he listen to me? Look at me? Was he really "present" in the examining room with me?

So even a very short visit can seem longer than one that took more time (by the clock), if you simply give the patient your full attention for at least part of the visit.

You benefit also, because putting full attention on your patient maximizes the stream of visual, auditory, tactile, and olfactory information you're getting. When you look—*really look hard*—into your patients' faces and eyes, you may glimpse there the answers to many clinical questions.

4. **Sit close.** If appropriate, **touch your patient**. Psychologically, patients experience us as distant and uninvolved if we keep too far away from them physically. From closer in, you'll also see, feel, and smell more, which sharpens your clinical impressions and diagnoses. And we don't always have to tower over our patients—it can make them feel inferior at a time when they may already be feeling one down. Sit.

You know about the research showing that infants who are touched and stroked grow up healthier and more confident. This same principle applies to your adult patients, who need to feel braver and more confident. This isn't just corny stuff; it's the difference between a more successful and a less successful clinician.

A patient who went into the hospital with a suspected MI felt frightened and alone. None of the doctors or nurses touched him. Finally a technician, while doing his echocardiogram in the ER, sat on the gurney, touched him, and leaned on him casually during the procedure. Her warm human contact, calmness, and good spirits were reassuring to him at a very basic level, he told me; for the first time on that frightening day, he was able to relax.

There's a good reason health care staff are privileged by society to touch strangers physically. People who come to us need reassurance and support as often as they need medication or a procedure, and few things are as comforting as the touch of another human. Touching also makes the bond between us and our patient closer, no matter how brief the visit. Sitting close and touching take no extra time, while both we and our patients benefit greatly.

Some obvious exceptions: touching people sensually, and touching disturbed or paranoid patients. The laying on of hands used to be a sacred healing ceremony, to be performed only by those who were pure of heart, etc. If touching people makes you nervous, or if you're in a lousy mood and you're probing and squeezing too hard, lay off instead of on.

5. **Allow a (brief) unstructured moment.** It's almost impossible to teach this maneuver to beginning residents. They come to patient interviews with a list of questions in their minds which they feel they absolutely must ask; the patient usually has a completely different agenda. Or as the doc said as he auscultated the chest of a patient who was trying to tell him something: "Quiet! I can't hear you while I'm listening!"

If we don't give our patient a chance to get on the air with their own program for at least a moment, she starts feeling ignored and not listened to, and eventually clams up. Usually, the physician then misses some crucial information completely—and trashes the relationship.

---

**"Do not interrupt us again!"**

Neurologist J.M. Charcot
(Speaking to a patient while on rounds)

---

If you're too rushed to fit it in anywhere else, at least ask near the end of the interview, "Anything else?"—then pause half a beat. The patient may have nothing to add, but she senses that she's been listened to, and given the chance to bring up whatever is bothering her. This takes only a second or two, but makes a definite impression.

Once I was present when the poet Darshan Singh was being examined by a number of specialists at a major medical center. One after another, each specialist performed their examination procedures. Finally, a cardiology fellow asked if she could listen to his heart. "Just imagine that!" the poet said delightedly, playing on the words. "All these specialists…but she's the only one who has wanted to listen to my *heart!*"

6. **Always say something positive and praiseful.** It's amazing how few physicians regularly perform this tiny kindness, which costs nothing and makes all the difference to our patients.

Every human needs a word of praise, approval, reassurance, or comfort. After you've questioned your patient, checked the data, and probed their anatomy, it's the perfect moment to say something that will make them feel better about themselves and about their condition. Our patients may at times be helpless, but they need never be hopeless—if we are humane.

Praise their body ("How come you're 70 and still have black hair, Mr. Smith? What's your secret?"), or just reassure them about what you guess is worrying them ("You know, for someone who's had diabetes as long as you have, your eyes look quite good, Ms. Green"). You can always find one or several things to say about them that will be received as sincere praise or good news about their physical selves (patients fear being criticized or receiving bad news).

> ❝The deepest principle of human nature is the desire to be appreciated.❞
>
> William James

Start doing this every time you see a patient; make it a habit. It takes no extra time, leaves your patient feeling great—and at the intimate interface of body and mind, good feelings can help promote better health. Isn't knowing that fact part of being a successful physician?

7. **Psychosocial talk.** Research shows the one type of physician communication that patients find most satisfying is "psychosocial" talk about function and feelings.[5] ("Are you still able to open jars and cans?" "How worried are you about what that chest pain may be?") It's vastly more popular with patients than the strictly "biomedical" style of most physicians: lots of diagnostic questions and instructions on regimen, but little interest in how they're actually functioning and feeling.

It's unfortunate that when physicians have to speed up their visits, psychosocial communication is the first thing to be eliminated. Very few docs now use it (only one fifth of the number who use the biomedical approach), but patients definitely prefer it, and research indicates that the psychosocial-style visit actually does not take any longer than the biomedical type. Consider moving toward this style of communicating with your patients.

8. **Avoid unprofessional remarks.** Patients are almost painfully sensitive to what we physicians say, and how we say it. Often they'll totally misunderstand a careless or ill-timed remark, and never return to tell us about it. Of course—especially during a procedure—never say, "I certainly hope this works" or "Uh-Oh!" or "Whoops!" Sounds silly? It happens.

Pray with Me

A physician friend of mine recently went in for endodontic surgery. Anxious, drugged, and slightly confused (like most patients), he was hypervigilantly listening for any signal that not everything was going right. To his chagrin, about an hour into the procedure, he heard the dentist say to his assistant, "Now let us pray."

Let us pray! My friend's worst fears were realized. Thinking something had gone seriously amiss with the surgery, he had a moment of blazing panic and was ready to jump out of the chair. Only by sheer force of will was he able to contain himself.

Just then the dentist repeated to his assistant, "OK, now let us spray again."

There's a pretty good chance that patients don't fully understand our instructions to them—after all, they're nervous, preoccupied, maybe embarrassed and confused. Asking, "What is it you don't understand?" will save phone calls, return visits, and frustration on both sides.

9. **If you speed up, be sure to slow down.** You may have become fast and efficient at locating needed information, formulating the case, doing procedures, etc., so that you're going through your patient work at a high velocity and getting it done more quickly. That added speed will leave you time to slow down when it's appropriate and make direct human contact with your patient.

This is not just a matter of style. Patients value a moment of personal attention—no matter how brief—more than routinized medical service. What good is speeding up if you don't use some of the time you save for the most satisfying part of your work? At least be aware when you feel you should change speed for a moment, and slow down. It takes a bit of practice to get enough control of your velocity to speed up and slow down at will. Barreling through your day, always at top speed, can become a habit, and it annoys people.

10. If you cannot find time to slow down and listen, **train your staff to listen to patients' stories.** They will then become the priceless database of your patients' narratives, and can give you tips that will explain puzzling developments in a case that might otherwise take a lot of your time, effort, and expense to clarify.

They'll know which patient has stopped taking their meds, who's drinking, who's getting separated or having serious financial problems, etc. If your staff person is also bilingual, then her value in this area becomes pure gold.

## Be Aware of Self-Presentation

Studies show that patients have pretty definite preferences about, and reactions to, our physical appearance—for instance, to our apparent age (they prefer us to appear over 27, but under 65) and to our dress (white coats and ties preferred for men).[6,7] We rarely think much about our personal self-presentation.

### The Doctor's Bag

Once each year our med school scheduled a Saturday morning session, conducted by a salty former military surgeon, which was the only formal training we had in how to present ourselves publicly as physicians. Though this session was not required, and no credit was given, the locker room buzz had it that this lecture was absolutely not to be missed, so we all showed up.

I still remember the surgeon's opening. He asked one of us to bring up the little black bag we each carried, and he just dumped out its paltry contents on the podium.

"Look at this piddling little bugger!" he roared. "You call this a doctor's bag? You're lucky if you can fit a sandwich in here! Your patient sees this little bag, he knows you're not serious.

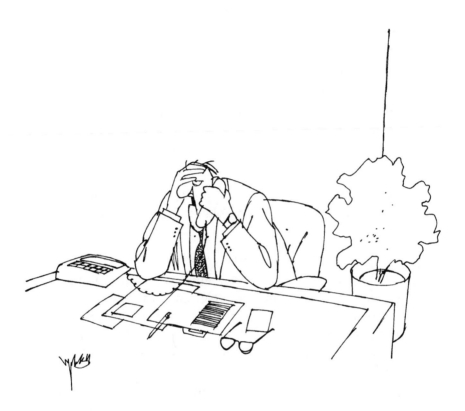

"Well I'm sorry I haven't come up to your expectations madam,…perhaps what you're looking for is a combination of Nostradamus, the Wizard of Oz and the staff from Chicago Hope…"

"Now here, ladies and gentlemen"—from behind a table he hauled out a heavy, scuffed bag the size of a big Pullman suitcase, overflowing with instruments, tubing, suture kits, gloves, needles, syringes, bottles, jars, slides, dressings, drugs, flashlights, sets of tools, spare batteries, handbooks, and God knows what else, and slammed it down on the podium with a triumphant *whomp!*—"Now here, ladies and gentlemen, is a real doctor's bag, a bag that says to your patient, '*This physician is a serious practitioner of the medical art!*'"

It was a little earthy, perhaps, but probably the single most practical and memorable lecture we ever had.

Try to **get some honest feedback** about how you come across to patients. You can listen more carefully to what's said about you, even notice what nicknames you're given. It will help a lot if you realize going in that every criticism you hear, no matter how unfair, contains some tiny grain of truth that you can learn from. There are also seminars and workshops you can attend to learn more about self-presentation.

Taking some time to **analyze your own interactions** with patients can help. When a relationship goes sour, what seems to have happened? Can you spot a pattern? Change the way you approach such patients? Can your staff help you understand what went wrong? (Ask them.)

One physician told me that he became imperious, patronizing, and arrogant toward patients during full-staff treatment conferences. It turned out that he felt resentment toward the non-medical and non-nursing members of his team, and tended to take this out on patients. Once he spotted this pattern, he was able to control himself better in conferences, and get more done in less time, with less friction.

## And Now, the Winning Clinical Style

Although most of us have had no formal training in precisely how to interact with our patients, it turns out that our style of practice is not only very important to them, but so crucial that using one preferred style can increase our patient retention by 100%.

In a recent study, two extreme styles of patient care were contrasted.[8] In one arm of the study, physicians treated their patients in the traditional, paternalistic way: They gave them no control over treatment, made unilateral decisions about treatment choices, and did not share responsibility with them for management. (This is still a pretty common way of dealing with patients, particularly among older physicians and physicians trained by old-style physicians.) According to this model, the doctor is the father, the nurse is the mother, and the patient is the child. This style was widely accepted in the days of patriarchal families, white male doctors, universal military experience, and public ignorance about medicine.

As you've noticed, those days are gone, and that style of patient care is definitely the wave of the past. Now our patients are educated, informed about medicine, and live in a nonhierarchical world of interactivity, from computers to talk shows. They're annoyed by the old, paternalistic style of medical care, and expect to be treated in the new, participatory style.

Basically, this newer style of practicing medicine has three crucial parts:

1. **Inform your patient constantly** and to the maximum extent possible about what you're doing, why you're doing it, what the alternatives are, what you plan to do next and why, etc. Do this in the most positive way possible, always using common sense about how to communicate information to your patient without alarming or confusing

her (not everyone enjoys seeing bones, tissue sections, etc. as much as we do).

This educational aspect of doctoring is becoming more important all the time and is a major departure from the days when we physicians purposely spoke and wrote to each other in Latin, called syphilis "lues," and generally tried to mystify everyone else. Informing our patients makes possible the other two facets of the participatory style.

2. **Share decision making** with your patient when choosing among indicated tests, procedures, and treatments. Patients want to make informed decisions in these areas—but studies also confirm that they really *do not* want to be included in your decision making about diagnosis ("Well, what do you think you have, Mr. Garcia, gallbladder or appendix?").[9]

   It needs to be said that it's hard for us to have a participatory style if we're cold, perfunctory, or machine-like in our approach. Some people in health care confuse ultra-fast, assembly-line, knock-it-out care with efficient care; that kind of care isn't really efficient at all. The most effective, satisfactory—and therefore most productive—approach requires some degree of sincere interest in your patient as a human being, and that means making some kind of human contact with them. If you're a successful physician, this is your intuitive way of working. We need to be careful not to let ourselves be forced into practicing superficially and mechanically in the name of efficiency; that kind of practice just ain't efficient.

3. **Share actual responsibility for treatment** with your patient. Patients want to be part of the treatment team these days, and should be given real responsibility for taking

meds, observing restrictions, doing self-care and exercises, etc. No fake, half-hearted lip-service ("Don't you worry now, we'll work together to get you well, Ms. Brown"). Today's patients have little in common with their parents ("Ohhh, doctor, I just trust you completely to make all the decisions"); they're knowledgeable, discriminating, and dedicated to being actively involved in their own care. This sharing of responsibility is less important if you're treating something acute such as an MI or a laceration. But increasingly these days we're treating chronic illness—which won't budge without lifestyle change (for instance, in the 70% of people who develop some form of hypertension). Many successful physicians now inform their patients point blank at the very first visit: "The outcome depends on you—in fact, this is going to be 'self-treatment.'"

## Participatory Pays

Now for the punch line: In the second arm of the study mentioned earlier, the physicians who used this participatory method of managing their cases had twice the patient retention rate of physicians using traditional, authoritarian approaches.[10] Also, patients who were able to ask questions, give opinions, and express treatment preferences had measurably better outcomes. So to keep our patients, and keep them well, we need to adopt this method of practicing.

For maximum efficiency and maximum patient satisfaction, consider combining the participatory model with the ten suggestions for optimizing the effectiveness of shorter visits; they will synergize.

Some physicians have complained to me that patients' respect for doctors and the medical profession is dwindling. Maybe we need to try changing our professional style to adapt to new social realities before blaming our patients for trouble in the relationship—and before they dump us for a more modern doc. Today's patients are different from those of a generation ago; as one patient put it, they want to know, "Where exactly is this bus going, and why is it going there?" So to keep more of our new patients, we'll have to meet their expectations and have enough faith in them to include them as our fully informed partners in the treatment process.

To put it more simply: These days, trust is a two-way street.

---

### Notes

1. A. Barra, "Arm and Leg Man," *Newsweek,* 28 October, 1996, 55–58.
2. D.M. Novack et al., "Physicians' Personal Perspectives May Influence Patient Interaction," *Journal of the American Medical Association* 278 (1997): 502–509.
3. "Patients Count Communication As a Major Factor in Measuring Quality of Care," *Resident and Staff Physician* 42, no. 2 (1996): 34.
4. Z. Neuwirth, "Physician Empathy—Should We Care?" *Lancet* 350 (1997): 606.
5. D.L. Roter et al., "Communication Patterns of Primary Care Physicians,"*Journal of the American Medical Association* 277, no. 4, (1997): 350–356.
6. D.K. Gjerdingen et al., "The Physician's Appearance and Professionalism," *Resident and Staff Physician* 36, no. 1 (1990): 65–70.
7. B. McKinstry and S.Y. Yang, "Do Patients Care about the Age of Their General Practitioner?" *British Journal of General Practice* 44 (1994): 349–351.
8. S.H. Kaplan et al., "Characteristics of Physicians with Participatory Decision-Making Styles," *Annals of Internal Medicine* 124, no. 5 (1996): 497–504.
9. R.B. Deber et al., "What Role Do Patients Wish to Play in Treatment Decision Making?" *Archives of Internal Medicine* 156 (1996): 1,414–1,420.
10. Kaplan, *Annals of Internal Medicine,* 497.

## ✦ 14 ✦

# Your Co-Workers Can Do More of Your Work

During my residency, I conducted a research study about what physicians, nurses, and patients each thought had made the patients well.[1] As expected, we physicians felt that it was our own medications and treatments that had helped the most.

Interestingly, most of the patients we surveyed disagreed; they gave most credit for their improvement to...nursing care.

That study opened my eyes: We physicians tend to under-appreciate the immense importance of our nursing and office staffs in our daily clinical work. Also, we pay almost no attention to the two billion nurse–physician encounters that happen every year. There is a fair amount of research and commentary on this subject in the nursing literature, but docs don't usually read those journals.

If we want to become highly productive physicians, we should stop ignoring this major part of our professional lives and start analyzing carefully our relationships with our staffs. They do an enormous amount for us, and they can do even more. For openers, they represent us to the rest of the world.

### How Well Does Your Team Represent You?

If you have a patient in the hospital, she'll be much more likely to judge the experience by her nursing care (which goes on 24 hours a day) than by the few minutes a day you spend with her. Which is fine, if you're confident about your team.

But a team is only as good as its weakest link. As you read this, someone else is dealing with your patients. How well do you know the nurses at your hospital (or who handle telephone calls at your clinic)—the ones who come on duty at midnight? How about the staff who float in over weekends and holidays? Would they be your first choice to represent you to your patients when you're not there? Are your nursing and office staff capable and motivated enough to be your eyes and ears, and to speak and act for you around the clock?

I call on corporations quite a lot, and I run into quite a lot of rudeness, coldness, and even cruelty from employees of companies that claim publicly to be "customer-oriented." My impression is that these employees must be unhappy with their work—satisfied workers don't act like that, not to customers, and not to patients.

So take a few moments here to think about your team; include everyone who works with your patients in any capacity, at any time. Are they fully competent? Do they work well with patients? With you? With each other?

### The Weak Link

Doctor T, a skilled gastroenterologist, had recently hired yet another new technician. While undergoing a procedure, one of Dr T's patients could not help noticing how inept the new technician seemed to be. Several times Dr. T had to remind her about cleaning an instrument, keeping some dressings in order, etc. Not only was the new technician clumsy and poorly trained, she made several unprofessional remarks during the procedure, and joked in an inap-

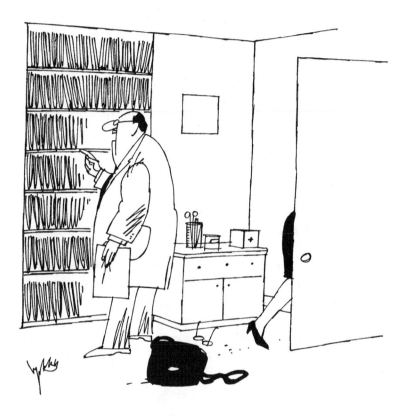

"...As my new office manager your first project is to copy
and re-code these patient records..."

propriate way with the patient. ("Do you mind having that sticking out of you for the rest of your life?")

The patient became understandably upset, and he decided on the spot to change physicians. As he was leaving the gastroenterologist's office, he asked the receptionist, "How come Doctor T has new technicians all the time? They don't seem to be fully trained."

"Oh, that's how he saves money," the receptionist confided. "Because they're untrained, he gets them for a lower salary."

At least in this case, it was a false economy.

## Leading the Dream Team

If you are fortunate enough to be the leader of an efficient and smoothly functioning team, you're already aware of it. The sensation of a well-oiled, hardworking, high-morale, medical or surgical team going at full throttle and optimum challenge is unmistakable. The work seems almost to be doing itself—the right instrument slaps into your glove at just the precise millisecond, someone has already hung the fluid or drawn the drug or found the data that you need before you can ask, and you're aware only of concentration, velocity, precision, singleness of purpose, punctuated perhaps by the occasional wry crack to keep everyone in good humor; it's a rush.

We've all had moments or hours or days when we worked with a team and it felt that way. If your day usually goes so well, be thankful. Sounds like you've got the dream team. You no doubt like and appreciate them a lot—don't forget to tell them that.

There are some minor disadvantages to having the best team around: You will be referred the toughest cases (try to negotiate with your team about taking on extra-difficult work), and other professionals may feel left out or envious (try not to boast or rub it in; be as helpful as you can to everyone outside the team). If you're just joining a crack team, it's probably best not to try to change the way they do things the first day; you could spend many weeks regaining everybody's trust. On the other hand, let them know early on that you have your own preferences and idiosyncrasies—but tell them in a pleasant way.

Of course, just when you think everything is going absolutely great, and you're sailing down the corridor on a cloud of success with everyone giving you the high sign and telling you that you're the best, that your team can treat the hardest cases in the world, etc.—that's when you should start counting the sponges and checking your malpractice coverage, because it often happens that clinical pride goeth before the clinical fall, and that's precisely when things will go wrong.

If you already work with the dream team, we'll just suggest some things you could do to keep everyone happy. But if you don't presently work with such a team, you'll want to consider seriously how you can help your staff move to higher levels.

## Good Teams Deserve Good Leaders

Getting maximum performance from teams is a talent as rare as hens' teeth, even among managers; and few doctors (or lawyers or CPAs, for that matter) are considered very good managers.

Since a great team is as important to our productivity and peace of mind as having the right equipment and technical skills, why do we physicians put so much stress on technical expertise in patient care, while we make no systematic efforts to optimize the way we function with our co-workers?

Some physicians don't want to work seriously on their relationships with their teams because they feel that being the leader of a team is their birthright, sort of like divine kingship. Other docs are just too busy doing procedures, and don't realize how much they could amplify their technical effectiveness by having better-functioning teams. Most of us honestly believe we're doing just fine, so there's no need for us to work on improving our teams. We're probably wrong. From what our co-workers tell me, we could do well to take another look. If we carefully analyze our relationships with our staff, and get some honest feedback, we'll learn a lot.

Maybe we feel that a nurse–manager or someone else with personnel skills and training should be responsible for optimizing our team's functioning. They can do the team leading, and we'll just practice medicine. This attitude can lead to problems for our patients.

### The Doctor Wore Black

When I checked into the hotel in Ottawa, I noticed my room number was 911, so I had a premonition there might be trouble. Sure enough, at about two AM someone phoned to say, "Come quick! The woman in 933 is having a heart attack!"

When I got to Room 933, I saw that I knew the occupant (we were both attending the same meeting); she was a high strung, anxious type, who might be having an MI—but who also might be having a panic attack. I started to ask her a few questions while unobtrusively checking her vitals.

Suddenly the hall door burst open and a flying squad of paramedics charged in at full tilt, shoved me out of the way and, without a word, proceeded to strip the patient, insert various tubes and needles into her body, set up a monitor, slap a mask on her face, etc. They worked with grim, robotic efficiency—and without wasting a second on history taking or examination. The patient, understandably, really did panic at this point, and began wildly gesticulating and fighting the mask, trying to breathe or talk. If she hadn't had an MI yet, she was at risk for one now.

Meanwhile, in one corner, completely uninvolved in the fracas, sat a young man in a black vinyl jacket and black pants. By his side was a small leather bag. He looked demoralized.

"That's the doctor!" I realized with an unpleasant shock, "and he's sitting in the corner, while his team scares the hell out of the poor patient. Great."

"Are you the physician in charge of this team?" I asked him, not too pleasantly (I don't enjoy seeing patients heedlessly mistreated).

He looked at me like I was speaking Inuit.

"Is this your team? Are you in charge here?" I asked again, because he hadn't gotten it the first time.

Slowly, comprehension dawned in his face, as if I had reminded him of something he hadn't thought about for a long time. "Yes, I'm the…physician," he said.

I went on to tell him that I was also a physician, that I was slightly acquainted with the patient, that there might be an element of psychological overlay in the case, and that I thought his team of wild men and women were possibly making things worse by jumping all over her. As the physician in charge, he needed to take over direction of his team.

This seemed finally to spur him to action; he stood up, gave some orders to control his people, and began to work up the patient—who, it turned out later, actually was having a panic attack, not an MI.

> That was a powerful lesson to me about how bad it
> can get for the patient when the person best qualified
> to lead the medical team simply gives up their respon-
> sibility.

These days, we physicians need to develop good leadership skills as much as we need to learn good diagnostic or surgical skills. No matter what people with vested interests may claim, it's still true that because of our traditional authority, broad and intensive training, and position of central responsibility, we docs are the best fitted to lead our health care teams. This is not an elitist opinion, but simple practicality: If not us, who else would you suggest for the job?

But more and more of our clinical work is done with and by others. Physicians whose practices lend themselves to having physician extenders find that a good assistant can increase productivity a great deal. Surveys report that 30% of us now work with physician extenders, but they're wrong—because everyone on your staff is a physician extender, everyone does some of your work. And, if your leadership and teamwork are exemplary, they'll do even more of it, and do it well.

You can no longer afford to ignore your central impact on your team's performance, any more than you can afford to ignore the outcomes of your technical procedures. If you **learn to excel at leading your team**, your future in medicine is probably assured. If you do not, you're missing a major opportunity to become much more productive; you're also missing some of the great joys of modern medical practice.

If I seem to be pounding this point over the head, it's because I've become convinced that every single one of us (including me) could do much better in using this third tool of our profession. In fact, if every physician who reads this section of the book takes it to heart and becomes more skillful at managing relationships, our entire profession will take a leap forward, and we can undo some of our recent setbacks.

### With Nursing and Office Staff, the Key Word Is "Help"

Take ten minutes some day to stand still and just watch nurses in action. It's an awesome sight. They seem to be genetically programmed to help everyone: patients, doctors, visitors, other staff, and each other.

Nurses report that they could help us physicians even more—and save us a lot of effort and grief—if only we would let them.

So to get more from them, try to **give your nursing and office staff more opportunity to be of help**. In fact, their biggest complaint about us is the same one we've already heard from patients: We physicians just don't listen to them. (Do you see a pattern here?) I believe that whenever a nurse gets frustrated enough to say about you, or any other physician, "He just doesn't listen!"—she means a lot more than the simple words. She's also saying, "He doesn't know how to work well with a team," "He doesn't respect us," "He's not working safe," "He refuses to accept our help," etc. So if you ever hear (or overhear) this being said about you, consider it to be a bright red light blinking on your dashboard; there'll be trouble up ahead if you keep driving without making some repairs to your relationships with your team.

### Success Secret

A few years ago a young internist of my acquaintance started practicing in a city that is notorious for having a surplus of doctors in his specialty. To my surprise, his practice has grown very rapidly, and he now has more patients than he can handle. I asked him what was the secret of his rapid success, in spite of so much competition from established practitioners.

"A lot of my new cases are referred by nurses at the hospitals where I attend," he told me.

"Yes, but why do the nurses refer patients to you, instead of to more established docs?"

"Because I talk to the nurses—none of the other doctors do."

Nurses try hard to flag us down and let us know things that they think will help us be more effective. We usually hustle through our workday without giving them our full attention and without taking seriously enough what they have to tell us about our patients, and our constant rushing makes us seem rude and inconsiderate. Do you have these symptoms of "rushing doctor syndrome?"

✦ You don't let nurses finish their sentences or reports to you.
✦ You schedule too many patients for the available time, so you have to go much too fast.
✦ You don't look at your nurses while they talk to you; instead, you read the chart, review the lab work, etc.

If you're a rusher (many of us are), think about this: If you can slow down long enough to listen to your nurses and form relationships, they will do more of your work for you—and then you won't have to rush!

So reinvest some of the time you're saving (by managing your schedule and knowledge base) into establishing better working relationships with your staff. Start by listening closely and attentively to what your nurse is telling you. Stop what you're doing and really *look* at her. This one act can change the quality of the whole relationship, just as it does with patients. Since you'll probably be the only physician around who listens like this, you'll get special help and consideration, as will your patients. And you'll learn a lot. Everyone will be more productive and live more happily ever after. Another win-win-win.

## Your Behavior Shapes Your Team's Behavior

Read that heading again, and let it sink in for a moment. It's what *you* do and how you do it that shapes the attitudes and habits of the people who work around you. This is a major attitude change, and may sound counterintuitive, but keeping it in mind will work like a charm to increase your team's productivity.

For instance, our actions can actively discourage priceless communication from our staff—priceless, because it can save our patients pain and risk, and us a lot of unnecessary trouble. A Nevada obstetrician told me this story: One morning he wrote an incorrect order, and his patient received an overdose of medication. When he asked the med nurse why she'd passed a dose that was clearly in error, her response was, "Whatever the doctor says, I consider it to be the word of God."

(Now, we might feel personally outraged by this event, even blame it on the nurse, insisting that she had ethical and legal obligations to question the order. But the point is that it happened, and such events are not uncommon. Recently a nurse at an East Coast hospital passed a fatal overdose of medication to a patient that had been ordered erroneously by a resident, and gave pretty much the same explanation.)

My obstetrician friend realized that all was not sweetness and light between him and his nursing staff, so he sat down with one of them to talk things out. She told him frankly that whenever nursing staff would call his attention to near misses (i.e., correctable errors) he had made, his response was to blow up at them. He would grumblingly correct his slips, but he acted so indignant that nurses felt bad about pointing them out to him.

Naturally, after a few scenes like this, they simply stopped catching this doctor's errors for him.

If our own behavior with nursing and office staff is anything like my obstetrician friend's, maybe we can correct it before anything serious happens. In fact, we might make it a general rule to **analyze our possible role in creating any misunderstandings or friction** between us and our co-workers. Some of us automatically consider every glitch to be someone else's problem, never ours. This means we're incorrect at least some of the time—and, worse, that we give up the opportunity to improve things by changing the way we handle situations with our co-workers.

From working with scores of different teams over the past three decades, I've become convinced that a physician can improve the behavior of her team, *if she makes a systematic effort to act differently herself.*

> Admitting we're wrong takes a lot of courage;
> admitting someone else is right takes even more.

What would have happened if my obstetrician friend had told the first nurse who caught a slip, "Thank you! You saved everyone a lot of trouble, and I appreciate it. In future, any time you think something looks funny in the chart or on the floor, I really do want to hear about it, no matter how rushed I am"—(errors are one exception to the "no interruptions" rule)—"in fact, I'd rather hear about ten things that might turn out not to be errors, and catch one, than have it the other way around."

He could also have discussed with his nurse how the slip might have come about, so that she could begin to understand more about his unique way of practicing, the thread of his clinical routines. This kind of exchange is priceless, because it allows your nurses to spot high-risk situations and prevent or neutralize your slips before any patient is put at risk.

And wouldn't it have been even better had he thanked and encouraged this nurse in front of the whole staff? News like that travels fast, and my obstetrician friend soon would have had every nurse on every shift devoted to watching his back seven days a week. Not too bad a trade for a few seconds of sincere humility and gratitude—yet how few of us do it!

## How Do We Doctors Get So Arrogant?

Although down deep we know that our nurses and office staff really are trying their best, and have our interests at heart, we can still be rude, blustery, and arrogant toward them. Some of us make our co-workers' lives less pleasant a lot of the time, and almost all of us do so some of the time. In fact, in a recent survey 1,800 ICU nurses listed interpersonal conflicts as their greatest source of stress; nurse–physician conflicts were reported to be the most frequent and most intense.[2]

Here's a lineup of some unpleasant physician characteristics our co-workers notice in us. Think carefully about each item to see if it sometimes applies to you.

1. That word *arrogance* comes up constantly whenever our staff describe what they find most unpleasant in us docs. We "act superior," "play God," "don't pay attention" to their input, and insist we "know better."

Whether we are in truth superior beings, who do always know better, and who really are God, is beside the point—people find this behavior obnoxious. Even at the opera, the days of the prima donna are over.

Probably all of us can remember being called arrogant at some point in our career. Yet we don't hear much about arrogant veterinarians or arrogant petrochemical engineers. So what's going on? Why so many arrogant docs? We probably come by our arrogance the same way my college buddy Tony came by his mustache.

### Tony's Mustache

Only 19 when his father died, Tony inherited a seedy Manhattan hotel staffed by a rough crew of bellmen, cooks, busboys, etc. These wiseguys considered him young and inexperienced, and were not about to listen to anything he said.

Until Tony grew a huge black handlebar mustache, fairly bristling with macho authority. That mustache did the trick: It made Tony look older and more masterful—and I think he also believed his own public relations! Anyway, from then on he was able to manage his hotel.

Most likely we grew our arrogance, like Tony's mustache, when we were thrown into the ER, clinic, or OR at a fairly tender age. A critical case arrived, and someone turned to us and announced, "Doctor, you're in charge now." We suddenly found ourselves the nominal leader of a team of seasoned workers who'd been doing their stuff for years or decades. Like the battle-hardened grunts of a war-weary platoon, they probably were praying under their breath that the newly minted first lieutenant (you or I) at least wouldn't get anyone killed.

In such a situation, it was inevitable that we adopted an air of total and instant superiority, as a defense against our realization that we didn't have a clue. Later, at some point in our training, our clinical experience and knowledge kicked in, we actually did become mature, competent physicians—and we didn't have to act arrogant any more.

Except by then it may have become an unfortunate habit. Arrogance is hard to shake. With a hot, unwelcome flush, it will surface in even the most mellow and seasoned physician when he feels directly threatened in his judgment and authority (that's how he got arrogant in the first place), or seriously stressed, or just exhausted.

In such situations it may help if you stop, look, and listen: *stop* what you're doing, really *look* at the people you're interacting with, and *listen* carefully to what they're saying. You'll **realize they're on your side**.

Usually we're in such a major hurry to get our very important clinical tasks done quickly and accurately that anyone who slows us down, questions our authority, or distracts us will provoke us to frustration, anger, or even abuse. This chain of events is so common that we don't notice it in our daily routine; it just seems to be part of being a doc. In fact, some practitioners have told me with straight faces that arrogance is a positive characteristic, and by being unpleasant they keep people from bothering them or going against their wishes.

Yet many excellent and productive physicians are able to get superb work out of their teams without friction and hurt feelings. These physicians seem to have a different attitude toward their coworkers. Instead of seeing their staff as getting in the way, their mantra goes something like: "Everyone here is trying to help me get my work done; they may at times be slow or inaccurate, but they are trying to help. Instead of blowing on them, therefore, it makes more sense to facilitate their helping me, by letting them know I appreciate their help, and by communicating to them how they can better be of help."

Try changing your own attitude in this direction. It helps—both you and them.

2. Arrogance is much more common in young docs, but at the other end of our career, as we grow older and slower, we may adopt the myopic, cranky habits of the *old curmudgeon*. This persona also keeps people tiptoeing around us, and it covers up an uncomfortable realization for any physician: that we're past our prime and losing some of our youthful powers.

The subject of the aging physician would take up a whole book, but suffice to say that 30 or 40 years of practice change a physician, and bring special pleasures—and also problems. Interestingly, learning new things need not be one of the problems: Research shows that older people can learn quickly (but are not as motivated to do so). So it's more a question of attitude than of aptitude.

Anyway, being a curmudgeon is a short-lived problem, relieved either by updating our skills, downsizing our practice—or retiring.

3. *Money-hungry.* Medical practice has been defined as "science plus emotion." Our co-workers and patients are not insensitive to our real inner feelings; if our ruling passion is greed, they pick up on it. As more and more doctors earn less and less, this may turn out to be a self-correcting problem, since there are so many easier ways to make lots of money than getting a lengthy medical education. It is part of being a professional to be paid for our skilled services, but it is unprofessional to sacrifice serving our patients to stuffing our pockets. Want to get rich quick? Consider a different line of work.

4. *Paternalistic, male chauvinist.* Some older male docs still call their staff "girls"—as in "I'll have my girl call your girl to set up an appointment." Or we introduce a mixed group to a patient: "This is your physician, Doctor Black, and your nurse, Joan."

These habits seem minor, but they signal that we don't consider our female staff fully equal members of our team. After 30 years of struggling for job equality, women still make up 96% of our nursing staffs, while four out of five physicians are male.[3] We need to be more sensitive about this issue and how we handle it; we should not brush it off as irrelevant to our work. Nurses, especially younger nurses, now wish to be treated as equals. E-q-u-a-l-s. They are serious about this, and they expect to be taken seriously. They may overlook much of our habitual paternalism, but they should not have to.

On the other hand, some nurses trained in countries with traditional cultures have told me they really don't mind this difference between doctors and nurses, and consider it an advantage: The patient needs to feel someone on the team is first-name approachable, and that turns out to be the nurse.

It's probably better not to take anything for granted: **Ask your staff what they prefer to be called**, and call them that. It may open up a dialogue on paternalism, if it's a problem—and asking the question will show you're interested in what is important to them.

5. Publicly bawling out or otherwise *publicly embarrassing staff*. Never a good idea. I did this recently myself (I can't walk on water, either), and felt lousy for days afterward—not to mention the fact that I permanently crippled a perfectly good and productive working relationship.

6. *Abusive, mean, and cruel*, taking out our own anger and frustration on staff. Here's a nasty little shock: In a recent survey of 350 nurses, 66% of them said they had been verbally abused by a physician in the past few months.[4] This is inexcusable and unprofessional behavior. True, we were probably abused during our training—85% of medical students reported "mistreatment or harassment" in a recent survey.[5] And that was inexcusable, too. Abuse is not an efficient teaching technique in the long run, and cruelty is among the lowest forms of interpersonal behavior. If you've been abused somewhere along the line, remember how bad you felt—and don't pass it on.

Docs can fall into subtler forms of abuse without even realizing it. Because of our education and personalities, we often tend to have a cutting, sarcastic sense of humor. This may go over well with colleagues, but nurses (who have different training and sensibilities) may misunderstand our barbs, and feel hurt. Save it for the OR locker room. Also, don't make remarks about nurses' weight or other physical imperfections. Even if you mean to be helpful, they resent unsolicited medical advice.

If you think about it, there's no good excuse for making others miserable. And the supposed end—getting more work done faster—never justifies the means.

### Are You Sure You're Not on the Doctor-From-Hell List?

Study the doctor-from-hell list one more time, and be really honest: Could any of those characteristics—arrogance, abusiveness, paternalism, etc.—apply to you? Often? Sometimes? (If you really think none of them *ever* apply to you, you're probably not being totally honest and self-aware.)

One quick way to get your eyes opened: **Start a conversation with your nurses about whether you are arrogant**, paternalistic, abusive, etc. I guarantee you'll get some new and astonishing insights. One caveat: Becoming acutely aware of how you make other people uncomfortable by your own behavior can be very uncomfortable for you—but that discomfort means you're starting to change for the better.

Only you can decide. If you will take time to analyze your own self-presentation, and also get some candid feedback, you'll probably want to make the effort to improve. My opinion? All docs would like to be good with people, and we can all do better. If I did not think we can change how we treat others, I never would have become a psychiatrist.

In general, if you try to **stay alert to the powerful effects that your words and actions have on the people around you**, you'll automatically start to change. If you do this for a while, you'll notice a difference in the way people react to you, and also in how much more smoothly and efficiently your work is getting done.

 **Exercise 14–1** During an entire working day, observe what you say and how you act toward co-workers (nurses, office staff, techs, OR staff), colleagues, et al. Try to be somewhat objective about how you're coming across to others, and use this benchmark: "Would I like to be talked to (treated) this way myself? Would it make me feel more or less like helping?"

Decide whether you need to make some changes in your approach. Start making them, and keep at it (it can be slow work).

But we need to do more than just quit annoying our co-workers. Let's turn to some positive suggestions for improving our teams.

**Notes**

1. M. Zaslove et al., "The Importance of the Psychiatric Nurse," *American Journal of Psychiatry* 125 (1968): 482–486.
2. D. Green, "Reduce the Stress of Calling the Physician," *American Journal of Nursing* 97, no. 9 (1997): 49–51.
3. Green, *American Journal of Nursing*, 50.
4. T. Begany, "Do You Get the Respect You Deserve?" *RN* 58, no. 5 (1995): 32–33.
5. D.C. Baldwin, "Student Perceptions of Mistreatment and Harassment during Medical School," *Western Journal of Medicine* 155 (1991): 140–145.

## ✦ 15 ✦

# From Scream Team
# to Dream Team

Some of us walk around muttering, "My team would be so much better if only those other people would change." Aldous Huxley said you can change only one corner of the universe: yourself. And we're not likely to get all new people to work with.

Because in medical school we receive zero formal training in the crucial skill of leading and managing a team, most of us are better at working alone, or at giving orders. During our residency, because we moved so fast through so many teams, it didn't matter if we weren't getting along with someone—we'd be leaving soon enough. We never got the experience of working with the same people over years or even decades. Now that we're mature practitioners, we can vastly increase our productivity if we perfect these skills and upgrade our own teams.

### How to Help Your Team Work Better

First off, don't expect your team to change overnight. Half-day "team-building seminars" are usually baloney. It takes months for habits, attitudes, and relationships to change. But they *will* change.

> **"Rome wasn't built in a day—but Rome was built."**
>
> Anonymous

When your team eventually achieves a high level of functioning, you'll feel it. Among other things, a good team:

✦ helps you feel more joy in your daily work
✦ cheers you up when you're down
✦ keeps you from burning out
✦ does a big portion of your work for you
✦ handles problem people (inside and outside the team) without being asked
✦ keeps you updated on news and information you need
✦ generally makes your workday wonderful

Physicians with high-functioning teams have told me they barely have to strain at all to get things done: Their team produces at a very high rate with a minimum of intervention from them, and most of the time they only have to touch base with their people regularly throughout the workday. These physicians have told me it's a very satisfying experience to look around the workplace and see their whole team working smoothly and effectively helping patients.

Social scientists use the term "situation awareness" for this kind of team function—everyone on the floor somehow knows where everyone else is at every moment, and all the work and all the hand-offs are getting done at the right moment in the right sequence, without friction or wasted effort, almost telepathically. When your team is working like this, all your tools—time, knowledge, and relationships—are meshing and synergizing for super-efficiency and maximum productivity.

Systems analysts dream of designing systems that can make the work flow this smoothly. But it's not a matter of human engineering or ergonomics or critical pathways or skillful delegating (though these can help). It's more organic than those mechanistic devices. High-level teamwork is conscious, capable human beings doing their best at what they do best, and doing it even better together.

This kind of teamwork is not just the result of team members' years of individual training and experience. If you want productivity like this, you have to be willing to make careful and continuing investment over time in your relationships with the people you work with. Here are some suggestions for helping your team be the best, from physicians who feel that their teams work efficiently and productively. Some of these ideas you may never have seen in writing before, and some may seem to you to be petty or impractical. But they work, so give them a serious try—and see if your own team doesn't start to improve.

1. **Set a prestige example, and set the pace.** You can't expect your team to work hard and smooth if you work lazy and rough. If your team is an orchestra, then you're the maestro. They're watching you for clues about how to work well together. So set a high standard...for yourself.

Good clinical work has the qualities of good music: tempo, rhythm, virtuosity, harmony, invention. In the OR, the surgeon literally has to set the rhythm of everyone's work. Some surgeons do it with music (Denton Cooley dissected to country and western). If things get out of sync during a procedure, surgeons have told me, it's important to pick that up early, use self-talk and confident nonverbals to radiate coolness and optimism, and not show anxiety or frustration. Thus, the best surgeons control the level of their teams' morale in the OR to improve outcomes.

Since you're setting the tone in any team, try to follow all of the next eight suggestions closely, and your staff will follow your prestige example.

2. **Think about your audience.** Every time you write or give an order, make a request, or ask a question of your staff, think

quickly, "How will this affect the people I depend on to get my work done?"

Yes, you can probably get away with writing illegible, unnecessarily complex, or difficult-to-execute orders. Yes, you can bark every time you talk to your staff, and they'll probably grit their teeth and put up with it. You can probably do lots of nasty things for a long time, and get away with them—but your co-workers will quietly resent your inconsiderate behavior, and eventually it will trip you up.

---

**"Empathy is a practical competence."**

Peter Drucker[1(p.118)]

---

Listen to the tone of your own voice when you're communicating with staff and colleagues. Do you notice a hard little edge of "Gotcha!" that creeps in when you're correcting or instructing someone? You may know a lot more than they do, but if you pounce or preen, people come to dread your superior knowledge instead of admiring it. Consciously train your clinical voice to be sweeter (including that crucial first instant when you pick up the phone and say, "Doctor Green here!"). Successful physicians have suggested that if you think for one second about your people before you speak or act (or even better, first inquire what would work best for them), they'll reciprocate this tiny human decency one hundredfold by making your work easier, smoother, and faster—and by doing a lot more of it for you, without being asked.

Several nurses have also mentioned to me that they very much dislike our cursing in front of them, especially using the "F" word. Not professional, and not necessary.

3. **Include everyone.** Your team is already working to meet your needs, but have you ever thought about whether everyone

on your team feels that their own needs are on the agenda, too? Try to find out what others want from the work. Make sure no one, including the custodian (who else will tell you whose pills are under their bed?), feels overlooked, left out, taken for granted.

Don't regularly take sides with any single faction in your team. If someone is an enemy of one of your friends, they can still be your friend, and you'll be the bridge between factions. Avoid hanging with just one clique, even inadvertently. Naturally, there'll be some people on your team with whom you feel you have more in common—but make some effort to give your time and attention equally.

A lot of the banter that goes on among mixed staff is sexual in nature; usually it's joky and innocent, but occasionally it's not. I'm sure some supervisor way back in your training warned you about the perils of mixing sexual relationships with work relationships, or else you've had to discover them on your own. Both staff and patients actually expect (and respect) that subtle but definite aura of professional distance we keep.

Don't gossip (no matter how juicy); stay above this popular but unprofessional pastime. Either be silent and don't participate, or gently remind people there's work to do. To join in gossip about other practitioners is particularly tempting, but it's also particularly unprofessional, so it makes people lose respect for you.

But having a chatty or gossipy person on your staff can be an advantage, if you encourage them to channel their natural talkativeness into encounters with your patients. While you personally don't want the distraction of small talk, worried patients welcome it—especially during a painful office procedure (call in your chattiest person to distract them), or while they're waiting for you to catch up on your schedule.

Backbiting is to be avoided by everyone, always. Talking negatively about someone who isn't there is basically deceitful. It will inevitably get back to the victim, who won't appreciate it, and it can have unexpectedly unpleasant consequences.

## The Joy of Backbiting

Dr. X and Dr. Y had been feuding for years over some ancient misunderstanding that they had never been able to settle. One of them started talking badly about the other in the nursing station one evening, and other staff joined in:

"Dr. Y is really not very professional," said one nurse. "He's rude to us a lot of the time."

"You know, I also have my doubts about his clinical judgment," said Dr. X about his colleague.

"And I have to cover for him a lot with his patients," complained a second nurse. "He really treats them badly sometimes."

A third nurse, who didn't even know Dr. Y, took all this in. Later that evening the hapless Dr. Y arrived to see his patients, and asked this nurse for a report.

"Do you really want to know how they are, doctor? Are you sure you even want to hear about them?" she asked with burning sarcasm.

Dr. Y was shocked by the nurse's sudden and unwarranted attack on him—and so was she. It took her some time to realize that her negative reaction to Dr. Y had no grounding at all in reality; her mind had been prejudiced by the backbiting session earlier that evening.

Later, she learned firsthand that Dr. Y was an able practitioner, even though Dr. X personally disliked him.

4. **Woo 'em.** Unless you're a movie director, the age of barking orders pretty much ended around the time Saigon fell. Every worker now expects to be given a sensible reason for doing things (especially hard or nasty jobs). The more sincere gratitude and courtesy you can show to all, the better. Smile at everyone. Be charming. It costs nothing, it takes no extra time, and it works wonders.

Small personal gifts from you are also treasured by your co-workers. For some reason, nurses love being given those little pens, notebooks, and other knick-knacks that drug salesmen give out to doctors.

Cultivate a better sense of humor. If you tend to the dour and grouchy, try to see the hilarious side of things. When you're working side by side with people in a tough situation, a gentle wisecrack can relax everyone fast. The absolutely best teams I have encountered in medicine seem to spend at least part of their workday laughing together. Laughter, it's claimed, boosts your immune system, so everyone will also be sick less—and automatically more productive.

---

Try especially hard to be pleasant on Monday mornings, so you don't ruin someone else's whole week with a sour remark.

---

Show some empathy...for your staff. If they're sad and miserable, share a little of it; if their youngster just made quarterback of his high school team, share their joy and their pride. Just because we're efficient doesn't mean we stop being human.

5. **Give them all the credit when it's due...** Craftspeople know when they've done a good job, but they still love hearing about it from you—in public, preferably. Praise builds your

people's confidence, so they'll undertake more and more skilled work on their own, making you and your team more productive.

While being generous with sincere praise, don't hog the credit for any successes. Let others say how great you are (they probably will, if you praise them first, but that shouldn't be the reason you praise them).

However, if things go wrong, always step up and take the blame yourself, and protect your team—you're gonna get the blame later, anyway.

Public praise is usually a good idea, but also keep in mind that there are some nurses and other staff whose still waters run deep; they like to work quietly in the background, and may be embarrassed if you praise them publicly in front of their co-workers. But they do love praise, so let such individuals know privately, by your tone of voice or a smile, that you personally appreciate their excellent work.

6. **...and even when it's not due.** A powerful team technique: Praise someone when they know they don't really deserve it, and next time they *will* deserve it, because they'll try like crazy to live up to your praise. This is counterintuitive, but it almost always works.

7. Repeat: **no public bawling out**. I suspect that many people underwent catastrophically painful early childhood experiences of being publicly punished or embarrassed; I see it happening in the supermarket, when an overwrought parent jumps on their child for dropping a jar of jam or some other minor mishap. If you're unlucky enough to publicly castigate someone with this kind of history, you can inflict major psychological pain—and earn a lifelong enemy to your professional success.

In fact, try to make it a rule: no bawling out at all. (But we're all human, and don't whip yourself if you fail to hit the 100% mark on this; it's an ideal, a target.) Since fear, shame, and embarrassment really don't motivate anyone for very long, why spread them around your team? Seasoned people know when they've screwed up, and they don't need you to remind them. If you think someone really needs a talking-to, be professional: Say it in private, when your temper has cooled. Or let someone else do it (personnel micromanagement is not the best use of your time).

8. **Get the best people and hold on to them…** Do everything possible to get good people to come and work with you. Not only will they be a joy for everyone to work with, they'll know other good people, and they'll bring them aboard, and so on, making your team even better.

Good generally comes from good. Good doctors know other good doctors, good nurses know the best nurses, etc. Everything gets done better and more efficiently if you work along the informal networks of excellence that exist within the health care system.

9. **…until it's time for them to go.** No one is indispensable or irreplaceable. The best people grow and change and move on. Don't take it personally that they're leaving you. Wish them well, have some Chinese food sent in for everyone, and then get back to work. There's another good team up ahead for you, believe me.

Finally, whether you've worked together 30 minutes or 30 years, don't forget to say at the end, "It was good to work with you."

## How Nurses Judge Us

During a survey we asked nurses, "How do you judge a doctor? Is it by how many years of training we have, or where we did our residency? By our technical skills? By how well we handle patients? By how we interact with nursing staff?"

Interestingly, it was usually none of these. Most nurses told us they judge physicians by the same criterion: how we react under severe stress.

When the patient in ICU is coding, when all hell has broken loose in the OR, the ER, or wherever; when everyone else is freak-ing out or stressing out or bugging out, one person has to stand their ground, stay cool in the midst of the chaos, decide what has to be done, and do the needful.

That person is you.

Osler called it *aequanimitas,* and in his most famous address he exhorted young doctors to develop this virtue of courage under fire above all others.

### Not As a Stranger Shall You Greet Death

Doctor G was a newly minted assistant professor of surgery at a major medical center. He was considered a "comer": He'd published promising research, his clinical smarts were admirable, and his residents liked him.

Now it happened one day that a patient of his began to die. This patient had a severe cardiac malformation, and the fight to save him had been long and hard. At the last hour the team assembled at the patient's bedside; the young professor was there, and so were several residents, med students, and nurses.

Just as the patient gasped and gave up the ghost, the professor suddenly bolted out of the room and ran down the hall and off the floor, leaving the rest of the team to finish up. He just could not face the death of his patient.

Word spread like wildfire through the whole hospital: Professor G had run away. He'd lost his courage. He was chicken.

The professor's reputation never recovered. Every new resident, student, and nurse heard the story. It finished him. Within a year he had left to practice in another state.

Another story: Dr. L was a neurologist, but because he'd served at an isolated overseas air base, his surgical and medical skills were intact when he came to work at a community hospital. One evening a seriously ill patient coded. A line was inserted, but the victim started to choke from apparent laryngeal edema. One or two other docs tried to intubate her, but could not. There was panic in the air.

Just then Dr. L arrived and coolly began to intubate the patient. He did the procedure with apparent perfect calmness, moving crisply and efficiently. The panic subsided, and the intubated patient was whisked away to the CICU.

Word about Dr. L's coolness under pressure spread along the hospital grapevine. He was admired, congratulated, even offered the next rotation as chief of medical staff.

He lived up to his reputation, and served his patients well. Tragically, a few months later, he was dead of AIDS.

We still miss him.

Medicine is the most honest of all the professions. It can't be faked. No matter if we talk a great case, dress sharp, become rich, powerful, and well known—there always comes for every physician the private moment of truth: Will we act decisively to help our patient when he or she most needs it? *Aequanimitas* comes from training thoroughly, from having good models, from undergoing hard and humbling experience without being ruined by it, from living life deeply, from loving and being loved, and from something and somewhere beyond our usual physical existence that we can't easily describe. It is greatly admired.

## Helping Your Helpers

We've already talked about the advantages of training them yourself, but if you also **sponsor your staff at educational activities** (or get your organization to do so) they'll come back to you inspired and ready to work smarter. In the future, you all may be able to go together to training arranged for your entire team.

In these days of cost cutting and reengineering, no one can stand on ceremony any more. **Have your staff constantly cross-train each other** so everyone can do everybody else's job. Then, if the time does come to shrink your operation, you'll be in a much better position to make the change.

Also, **show some interest, and ask each person on your team some detailed questions about how they do their job,** the skills and the tricks of the trade they use. They'll be thrilled that you actually take an interest in how they do things. This will definitely set you apart from the pack, because the vast majority of us docs just take our co-workers—and the amazingly skilled tasks they perform nowadays—for granted. You'll also learn some valuable stuff.

Don't forget to **have your staff get training in efficiency-enhancing disciplines** like time management, if they haven't already. When they notice that you're serious about putting some of the suggestions from this book to work in your daily practice, they'll get the idea and start finding ways to become more efficient themselves. If they show some interest in becoming more productive, encourage them.

And we physicians don't have to stand on ceremony as much as we used to, either—although in general, we shouldn't spend our time being file clerks or custodians. An ER doc friend of mine won over the staff his first night on duty by the homely act of fixing a jammed door lock with a screwdriver from his car's tool kit so they could all get on with their work.

If you really want to freak out your nurses, go in tomorrow and ask, "What can I do to make your lives easier?" They'll be stunned.

Helping goes both ways, too.

---

**Note**

1. T.G. Harris, "The Post-Capitalist Executive: An Interview with Peter F. Drucker," *Harvard Business Review*, May–June 1993, 115–122.

## ✦ 16 ✦

# Your Colleagues: A Matter of Respect

In Part 1 of this book I noted that I'm also a student of physician productivity, learning from the thousands of physicians who have attended productivity seminars since 1993. And one of the most important lessons I've learned is that all physicians are outstanding individuals, who deserve a great deal of respect.

### Earned Respect and Learned Disrespect

We physicians are more alike than we are different, and every physician has several crucial things in common with every other physician. First, out of 400 people (more, in some other countries), only one had the desire, brains, talent, courage, and altruism to become a physician: you. Every physician has had to pass through the fires of discouragement, self-doubt, and sheer desperation—now thankfully forgotten—to make it all the way.

> "How necessary is the practice of Surgery to you? Would you die if you were not to do it?"
>
> Richard Selzer, MD[1(p.37)]

This may sound sappy, but it's nonetheless true: Each of us traded in our youth for the privilege of working hard for the rest of our active lives trying to ease the suffering of our fellow humans. We gave up a lifetime of undisturbed nights, restful weekends, and normal family routines. Until the day we finally retire from patient care, during every waking moment, no matter where we are or what else we're doing, there's always a little piece of our brain thinking about our patients, like an "instant-on" TV with a trickle of current running through it all the time.

For this continuous work and sacrifice, we probably don't get paid as well as our college classmates with the same amount of brains and stamina who became successful at law, business, or computers. We are, however, blessed with the reward of really good workers—more work!

Medicine is so peculiarly demanding that every practitioner sooner or later has to adjust to the fact that it's more than a job, a career, or a profession. It's definitely a vocation, in the old sense of that word: a calling. It chooses you, and there's not much you can do except pursue it, wherever it leads.

## Two Students

On a recent evening two college men came to visit our daughter. Sitting next to each other on the living room couch, they seemed similar in age, talent, and ambition. Yet one of them struck me as different: He burned with a familiar flame I could feel across the room, and whose intensity rekindled my own memories from 40 years ago.

He was a pre-med student, and totally, heedlessly obsessed with becoming a doctor. He would take an extra year at the university, study nine months for the

> MCAT, he would leave the country, do anything nec-
> essary—but he would become a doctor.
>
> For him, medicine will be a labor of love.

You'd think that since we're all sworn comrades in this wonderful undertaking called medicine, that we'd join arms and march
shoulder to shoulder into the broad uplands, etc. Not likely. We
physicians tend to be prickly critters, famously difficult in our relationships with other docs. So how did we turn out this way? Why is
getting along with all our medical colleagues such a rare skill?

Part of it is just the nature of our work: We're independent, self-
regulating professionals, and a great deal of our day is spent spin-
ning through our own solitary orbit. Even though we work in
teams, the heavy responsibility that we bear alone brings us to
assume a certain professional aloofness, so we tend to be self-con-
tained, even when we're with colleagues.

Also—and this is unfortunate—our attitudes toward other docs
get turned around during school and training. Competing with all
those other pre-meds was not conducive to chumminess. Then, if
we trained in a university medical center, we learned to look
down on the supposedly less-than-brilliant "PMDs" and "LMDs"
("private physicians" and "local physicians," respectively—as in
the chart note, "The referring PMD believed this patient had the flu
and failed to work him up for systemic lupus erythematosus,
etc.").

This attitude makes no real sense. We busy practitioners may
not have time or resources to do the kind of exhaustive clinical
work done at the best medical centers, but it turns out that a lot of
what we do is better. I've already mentioned how volume makes
some of us more skilled at certain procedures than any professor.
University medical centers co-opt and then develop innovative
treatments (laparoscopic surgery, lithium for mania, etc.) that
started in the boonies, with busy practitioners like you and me—

PMDs and LMDs. So we can drop the more-professional-than-thou attitude.

## Make the Effort to Reach Out

Also, heavy pressures from the new, competitive system of financing medical care are tending to split us off from some of our fellow practitioners. Many doctors are being told there are too many physicians in their specialties; this understandably brings out panicky feelings of survival of the fittest, devil take the hindmost, etc. Making generalists gatekeepers for specialists, surgeons' use of non-physician anesthetists, etc., have fired up old and new animosities among groups of physicians. With the rise of hospitalists and the lowering of reimbursements, more of us now spend our entire working day isolated in our office, never hanging out with our colleagues on the medical staff—if we still belong to a hospital medical staff.

How can we fight these centrifugal forces threatening to pull our profession apart? By investing effort into cultivating better relationships with other physicians. The key word here is *effort*. That means doing what may be a bit inconvenient for us: picking up the phone or driving to stay in touch, being aggressively friendly, asking our colleagues what they're worried about and whether we can help. Maybe because of stress, or because we're seeing so many patients, just being civil to each other is getting to be unusual. Recently a doc came up to me to say he had not forgotten my giving him a ride to a meeting when he was on crutches with a broken leg—six years ago!

Keeping up collegial relationships is something we didn't even have to think about back in the days when the hospital was a social center for docs. Then we had time for a leisurely chicken-salad-on-white-toast and two cups of coffee with colleagues in the staff dining room between cases, and we all talked with each other all the time. Those days are gone, so we have to go out of our way to reach out to other docs. Make it a habit.

## When We Look Down on a Colleague

A generalist friend griped about a partner who seemed to be ordering more consults than my friend thought was necessary. The physician to whom he was complaining put the situation into a new light when she remarked: "Of course he orders a lot of consults—and believe me, if you'd had the same problems with peer review that he's had in the past, you'd be ordering extra consults, too." More than criticism or backbiting, that partner probably could have used some unobtrusive coaching, role modeling, and friendly reassurance.

> **"No sin will so easily beset you as uncharitableness toward your fellow practitioner."**
>
> Sir William Osler[2(p.369)]

Maybe you're convinced that one practitioner in your medical community does work that is below your standard. But no doc is an island: You and he are in the same profession, and whatever lessens him lessens you, also. So if you decide to **work helpfully with your less skilled colleague** to see if he can improve over time, you'll be helping yourself—and his patients. It's an old saw that people perform at the level expected of them, so that practitioner just may pleasantly surprise you. I've personally been surprised more than once.

But just the weight of numbers dictates that there do exist a few physicians somewhere among our 750,000 colleagues who are incorrigible—though in many years of practice, I've seen only a few. To protect patients, we once in a great while have to bite the bullet and refer someone to peer review or to the department chair, if he is not receptive to our repeated help and suggestions.

On the other hand, someone who we at first think little of, given some help and some time, may grow to become one of our favorite colleagues. So it makes sense as a general rule to **give unpromising colleagues the benefit of the doubt**, until we're sure, one way or the other. But then we should act, and not slough the responsibility.

**Exercise 16–1** Think about the colleagues you regularly encounter. Is there one whom you consider to be having problems in his or her practice? Maybe their skills seem weak, or they're having trouble with relationships. Maybe they're a bit sour, or brash, or loud, or impulsive. Maybe you personally just don't much care for them, or maybe at some time in the past they've rubbed you the wrong way.

Try inviting that practitioner for lunch or coffee. Listen to them, see if you can understand their problems. If they ask you for advice, give it. Try to meet with them more than once, and see if you don't become friends. Gaining a friend and losing an object of dislike is a double gain for you, and another win–win.

### Fighting Each Other Weakens Us All

As medicine has become corporatized and competitive over the past five years, strains among physicians have been getting worse, getting us annoyed with each other and splitting us apart just when we really need to be hanging together.

We hear stories of docs who, under pressure from some megacorporation, sell out friends and partners to preserve their own high incomes (which are usually lost anyway, in the next round of discounting and disenrollment). Physicians have also told me they're disturbed to see a few practitioners, who perhaps cannot compete as well on skill or merit, taking the low but lucrative road of organizing cut-rate shops and then selling out. Physicians fighting like junkyard dogs over the bones of fees and contracts do not make a pretty picture.

### The Infamous Bombay Garbage Strike

During a week-long garbage collectors' strike in the subtropical city of Bombay, heaps of rotting, malodorous garbage began to pile up in people's yards.

Citizens in one part of the city handled the problem this way: Each householder just tossed the stinking garbage over their wall into their neighbor's yard, hoping to export the trouble. Unfortunately, their neighbors were doing the same thing—so everyone in that part of the city ended up with smelly piles of garbage in their yards.

In a different neighborhood, citizens decided to team together, taking turns collecting the garbage and hauling it to the dump. Naturally, that part of the city stayed clean and relatively sweet smelling.

The clear moral: When the situation stinks, don't try to dump on the other person; it'll just get worse for both of you.

Learning to pull together is a new need that some of us haven't had to face before. But if we're going to be successful these days—whether as a group, an IPA, a specialist care team, or a profession—we definitely need to know more about getting along with and working in harness with our colleagues. It's not just about getting referrals any more (although it is still true that a skilled and competent doc may get few referrals from her colleagues if she doesn't get along with them); it's about staying in practice.

> Practicing medicine these days is a symphony, not a solo, and each of us needs to know how to play our part with the rest of the orchestra.

The old-style, independent solo practice of medicine was like driving down an empty country road. You could slow down, speed up, stop, turn around, drive just about any way you wanted to, and it didn't much matter.

The new model of group and team medical practice is much more like driving on an eight-lane freeway. You're speeding along, bumper to bumper and side to side with a lot of other people, all locked together in a dense and intricate traffic pattern. You have to plan any change in speed or direction far ahead, very carefully, *taking all those other people into account*—or there could be a nasty pileup.

Unfortunately, the art of working closely and smoothly with all our colleagues is rarely practiced. It requires patience, flexibility, and some working knowledge of applied psychology. Fold down this page, and look at these suggestions again when you're having a falling-out with another physician in your treatment community:

1. Try to **look for the best in your colleague**, and to give her the benefit of the doubt if you're not sure.
2. Assume that most dustups aren't serious disagreements at all, but just the result of either bruised egos or simple misunderstandings—so **put your own ego on hold long enough to talk it through with your colleague**, and it'll probably get settled.

3. When we competed in med school, it was only because we each wanted make ourselves the best physician, the one who could help our patient the most. So you and your colleague are both fighting in your own ways for the same thing: to do what each of you honestly believes is in your patient's best interests. Once you flip the situation in your head and **realize that you're both trying to reach the same goal, even if your approaches are different,** you'll be friends again.

4. If hard words have been exchanged, **be the first to forgive and forget**, and you'll find the other doc is ready to do the same—then you can both quickly get on with the real work.

> Be careful who you practice with—not only because you'll have to handle some of the problems he creates, but because you'll inevitably pick up some of his practice habits.

Even if you're blessed with perfect colleagues, think about working harder at beefing up your panels, networks, and collegial friendships. There is real power in networking. (I'm not talking here about economically based networks of integrated health care organizations, but about your own personal network of colleagues.) You can get knowledge from your network, but you'll also get breaking news, support, advice, favors, job leads, validation. Be sure you give back in kind.

As hospitals and traditional medical staffs disappear one by one, we have to go out of our way to form and maintain wider networks of friendships and alliances. If you've ever been an officer or a noncom in the military, you know that enormous modern organizations actually function through informal but effective personal networks. People make fun of these I'll-scratch-your-back-if-you-scratch-mine arrangements, but they work; if they didn't, the submarines couldn't sail and the transports couldn't fly.

> This is the age of networks; those who can use their networks can control their future.

When you have good collegial relationships, you support and improve your profession, and its collective strength increases every physician's productivity—including your own. If we all get serious about working more smoothly with even one of our fellow practitioners, then the future begins to look a lot brighter. In fact, one managed care entrepreneur confided recently that he is scared witless by the prospect that some day we 750,000 physicians may stop our intertribal wars and start to focus as a unified force on the problems facing our profession.

## Artists and Doctors

It's said that all the great artists have a defining moment in their lives when they realize their work is not just a matter of individual effort—suddenly they become personally aware that they're practicing an art, something greater than any single individual, a collective undertaking that started long before they were born, and that will outlive their individual life.

And it's said that once an artist has this "Aha!" experience, their relationship to their work is changed irrevocably, and they can go on to become truly great.

Physicians and surgeons have told me they have experiences like this, too. At some point, usually a couple of decades into your career, you look around and notice that most of the older physicians you respected so highly are gone from the scene...and it occurs to you that you've taken their place. Now you're a stalwart of your profession, and it's your turn to carry forward the art and science you've been taught.

At that point you no longer feel that you're just an individual working and striving in isolation; you realize that you are a full contributing member of something far greater—an intrinsically noble mission to relieve human suffering, which spans the ages, and which plays a more or less crucial role in every person's individual history.

From the time of that realization, physicians have told me, they begin to see their work differently. The excellence of the entire profession begins to seem more important than individual competition or achievement, and transmitting wisdom and humane values to younger practitioners becomes a higher priority than fighting for yet more income or ever higher honors.

## Giving Something Back

At about the same time we realize we're part of something greater—Medicine with a capital M—we may also come to the conclusion that this profession has, on balance, been pretty good to us. Many of us trained at public expense, were guaranteed high-paying practices or salaried jobs from the start, and over the years have been provided first-class hospitals and clinics with expensive equipment and excellent staffs who take our orders—all given to us gladly, without question.

In spite of having definitely lost our hegemony in health care during the past 15 years, and having now to deal with powerful corporate monoliths we can neither fully comprehend nor influence, very few of us would actually change places with managers or businesspeople. Frankly, the privilege of helping our sick and injured fellows is too dear to most of us, and just amassing profit or power over others is not the road we chose. So it's no surprise that we want to give something back to society and to our profession. For most of us, this is just part of being a physician.

### The Resident Who Played Tennis

From the windows of the hospital where I trained, we could see the tennis courts quite clearly, several stories below. While we were sweating out 14-hour days on the wards, one particular resident was spending much of his day on the courts playing tennis, usually in his scrubs. There were always a few attractive nursing students hanging around watching him appreciatively, and now and then he would stop playing long enough to chat them up and make dates for later.

Watching from upstairs, we weren't so appreciative. We had to pick up a lot of his scut, and we probably envied both his coolness and his success with the women.

One day I complained to the attending: "Hey, what's with that guy? We're up here hustling our butts, while he's down there using his scrubs to pick up dates. What's the deal?"

The attending gave me an unforgettable answer. "Look, doctor, grow up. Over the years, you're going to find that there are two kinds of people in this profession: those who give to medicine more than they take from it, and those who take from medicine more than they give. And obviously"—he looked out at our friend on the tennis court—"he's one doctor who's going to take more than he gives!"

A surprising number of practitioners have mentioned to me that one of their great remaining pleasures is to **give some medical care freely**, i.e., free of charge or at a nominal fee, to indigent (or just plain hard-up) patients who need it. Even some appliances, medications, dressings, etc. get given away free.

There's no way to tell how much *pro bono* medicine is practiced in this nation of 50 million uninsured, where even patients with "good" insurance are finding it hard to gain access to a physician. Only each physician knows in her own heart how much care she gives away free. She doesn't have to account to anyone for it—it really is, after all, hers to give, if she wishes. And, like saying no in order to keep up our autonomy, giving our medical skills away seems to be our way of still being professionals, not just businesspeople. Maybe that's why it feels so good.

A renowned neurosurgeon told me that one of his favorite activities is dropping in on former patients around the world. He gets not a penny for these visits, but he says all patients need to feel they're not abandoned and alone—and making these visits has become the greatest pleasure of his professional life.

> **❝Well people can't really relieve the isolation of persons who are ill; only doctors can....Patients need a medical friend.❞**
>
> J.F. Drane, MD[3(p.84)]

In our residency years we may have learned to be disdainful or frankly insulting toward our elderly, chronically ill patients, calling them "gomers" or "hits," or worse. It does not cost us anything to be particularly nice to these victims of indolent, undramatic, but vexing conditions. Eventually, we'll succumb to the same kinds of conditions, and what goes around will probably come around.

A wise man once told me that the greatest desire of the sick and the elderly is simply to be listened to—yet no one does this. So whenever you or your staff can **take a few moments and just listen**, you're doing a great thing. Medicine is different from business in this way; taking the time to be human is actually more productive than rushing through our work, oblivious to the people around us. What gets produced? Saner, happier, more loving human beings. A few extra bucks at the bottom line cannot buy that product.

In our oath we promise to train without fee the son of any other physician. This promise translates today into millions of hours of attending, instructing, and mentoring given freely to our younger colleagues. Doctor means teacher; we naturally find great satisfaction in passing on what we've learned, as it was passed to us. The greatest gift we have to give is our experience, and that we can give freely. By training our new colleagues—and training them well—our profession has hope and a future.

---

**Notes**

1. R. Selzer, *Letter to a Young Doctor* (San Diego, CA: Harcourt Brace, 1996), 37.
2. W. Osler, *Aequanimitas* (Philadelphia, PA: Blakiston, 1932), 369.
3. J.F. Drane, *Becoming a Good Doctor* (Kansas City, MO: Sheed and Ward, 1988), 84.

## ✦ 17 ✦

# Serve Your Self

Giving to our patients is so ingrained in physicians' personalities that we sometimes count everyone else at the table but forget to count ourselves. Be sure to **take some time every day to...**

1. **Listen to Your Body.** Is it getting exhausted? Ill? Too old or worn out to keep up the pace you're setting for it? Are weekends or even long vacations no longer enough for you to feel rested?

Be realistic with yourself, because this is a tender area for most docs—we're Stoics, and we hate to admit we're tired or sick, or that our bodies can ever wear out. After all, we're docs—we don't get sick, etc. Yes, we do.

If you have hypertension, angina, diabetes, or any other illness, don't ignore it, don't treat it yourself, and don't procrastinate about getting the best treatment you can from the best people you know of. If you insist on ignoring the signs of illness or exhaustion, the weeks or months it takes to recover from a major blow will cost you much more in lost productivity than would a little preventive R and R.

Probably not a good idea: counting on your staff to tell you when you need to slow down. Too often these days, they need us to keep going constantly at top speed, so everyone's salary gets paid on time.

We may overload ourselves for psychological reasons. A surgeon friend from a western city told me about another surgeon who was killing himself, going faster and faster for longer and longer hours, trying to keep a huge practice open in spite of discounted fees and murderous competition.

"So why does he keep such a big, expensive operation going? Why doesn't he just use common sense and shrink it?" I asked.

"It's his ego."

Try to weigh the realities of your situation coolly and objectively, without getting nervous, and make the changes that make sense. Is it time to cut down? Slow down? Shrink your practice? Retire? Don't feel pressured to keep going like a 30-year old if you're 60; or 50.

Do you maybe just need a power nap every day after lunch? Don't smile—some older practitioners have confided that this simple measure (which they didn't usually tell anyone about) allowed them to extend their useful working lives by several years. Winston Churchill and George Bernard Shaw are just two of the high-achieving people who took daily afternoon naps to keep up their productivity.

2. **Listen to Your Mind.** How high is your stress level? Are you losing sleep (an early sign that you're redlining), losing peace of mind, losing your optimism and your oomph, burning out?

Since psychological stress comes every day, most physicians now find that they need to **do some preventive maintenance every day to neutralize stress**, and not let it build up. Whether it's playing a musical instrument, exercise, meditation, flying, sailing, relaxing with your family and friends, rebuilding your motorcycle, or whatever—it needs to be part of your regular schedule, because it's as important as anything else you do.

Using some of the time- and effort-saving suggestions in this book can help you lose some of your stress, but the suggestions about relationship management may help the most, because most of our psychological stress at work usually comes either from our interactions with other people, or from our own attitudes. Decide you just won't get upset any more over anything small: losing less than one hour of time or less than $150 just isn't worth banging on your arteries. Try alternating your tasks so you have some variety, and get all the collegial support you can. If your own efforts fail, professional therapy can help you feel much better (many of us have used it). In any case, don't sacrifice your own peace of mind to keep the ship afloat.

### The Drill Sergeant's Lesson

One 115-degree July afternoon in 1967, a dozen sweating physicians (including me) were crashing around in the middle of a Texas swamp. It was leadership training for newly enlisted Air Force docs who would be sent overseas in a few days, and the obstacle course was a grimly serious matter, in keeping with where many of us would be going (it was the height of the war in Vietnam, six months before Tet).

We made it to the last obstacle, a five-foot-high concrete wall. "All right, listen up, and carefully," said the intense young drill sergeant. "This wall is mined, and everything on both sides for five feet is mined. If you touch the wall, you'll blow up, and if you stay on this side, you'll be killed. You have to get your whole platoon over that wall, and you have to do it in under four minutes. The only equipment you have is this wooden pole. It's twelve feet long. Lieutenant, you've been doing a lot of talking this afternoon"—the drill sergeant tossed me the hunk of lumber—"now let's see if you can lead a platoon. Start...now!" and he blasted a shrill *phweet!* on his whistle.

Usually it's not easy for a dozen docs to agree on anything, but we'd been through a lot that afternoon, and were actually getting pretty good at planning and executing. The first idea was to use the pole to vault over the wall (but no one knew how to pole vault), then someone suggested swinging over one by one. Finally we arrived at a solution to the problem: Two of the strongest and tallest would anchor the pole on their shoulders on this side of the wall, we'd boost people up and they'd scamper over, and then they'd anchor the pole on the other side until we all got over.

It went like clockwork, until only two men were left on this side of the wall: myself and a surgeon from New York named Frank. He said, "Go ahead, Zaslove, I'll boost you up and you'll get over. If you hold it real steady from that side, I think I can swing up and get on it from here by myself."

But I had seen some John Wayne movies, and I knew just what I was supposed to do: "No way, Frank. I'll boost you up," I insisted, "and you get over first. I can make it from here. That's an order." Frank made it over easily, and they held the plank from the other side, but there was just no way I could steady myself on it, and it hit the wall. *"Phweet!"* went the sergeant's whistle, meaning the mines had exploded and the exercise was over.

We, of course, were jubilant. Everyone except me had gotten over, and we had worked fast, like a real combat team—pretty good for a bunch of myopic docs in boot camp. Maybe I'll get some kind of medal, I thought modestly, or an early promotion.

"Okay, you all did pretty good today," the drill sergeant told the other docs, "you worked fast, and you worked together. But you, Lieutenant Zaslove"—here

comes the medal, I thought—"You flunk the leadership course."

"What? Flunk? But we got everyone over, and we did
it fast—" I was truly indignant.

"Lieutenant, let me tell you something I hope you'll
never forget," the sergeant said. "You got everyone
over—but you sacrificed yourself. You were the leader
of this platoon. They were counting on you to lead
them from here. All you docs do the same damn
thing—you sacrifice yourself for others. That may
make sense to you, but it doesn't to us. Because, lieutenant, *you can't lead if you can't survive.* Wherever
they send you, I don't ever want you to forget that."

I never have.

If the stress just won't go away, there are always alternatives:
change your group, or your practice, or your specialty, or even
your career. Medicine is a good profession, but a bad obsession; a
noble pursuit, but not worth dying for. And severe stress can definitely kill you. Some young, hardworking docs I've spoken to recently have been quite honest about their intention to get out of
medicine after a few more years and go into computers or law or
whatever. It's unfortunate that promising young practitioners
(practitioners of any age, for that matter) are finding things so
rough that they plan to leave, but I can't fault their individual decisions. I hope some of them will read this book and change their
plans.

3. **Listen to Your Spirit.** For you, is medicine still a labor of
love? If so, you'll definitely find ways to keep practicing—even if it
means learning a new subspecialty, moving to a new state, or adjusting your financial expectations.

## Make Friends with Change; It's Not Going Away

Physicians tell me their biggest source of stress these days does not seem to be hard work (docs are all hard workers), but rather loss of control over their professional lives, reduced expectations, fear of the future—in a word, change.

It's easy to criticize new ways of doing things. We can say that laparoscopic surgery has these problems, managed care has those drawbacks, computers have so many glitches, etc., etc. In these pages I've fallen into that trap myself a few times—but I do not want to give the impression that significant change can ever be avoided or ignored. Distinguishing what must change in our practice from what must never change is crucial for our peace of mind. Take some time to think about it.

We've given many suggestions throughout this book for reducing your frustrations and annoyances by eliminating the ones you can eliminate, and managing the ones you can't. But change itself is now a permanent part of our professional lives; it's the result of gargantuan global forces (technologic, economic, demographic) that we can neither eliminate nor control. Here are suggestions from docs who are dealing with major changes:

1. Since we can't control or avoid change, that leaves us only one option: We have to adapt. So **don't procrastinate about dealing with change**. These days, physicians who dig in and stubbornly resist the inevitable seem to be the unhappiest and the most stressed. Remember how upset we all were a few years back about Medicare paperwork, DRGs, etc.—changes that we've now more or less adjusted to?

2. Rather than wasting time and emotional energy looking back to the Golden Age of solo fee-for-service medicine, try to **look ahead**. To analyze your situation, to **become aware of what's coming**, allows you to **think pro-**

**actively**, and recognize those changes that are unavoidable—and positive.

3. Making sure you **hang out with younger docs** has already been mentioned as a way to benchmark your clinical skills, and being with younger people in general (including kids) can actually help you adjust to change. They're the ones the changes will affect the most, and we can better understand new trends when we see how young people react to them with confidence and trust in the future.

4. Do a flip in your mind and **see change as an opportunity** instead of a loss (it's both, but why accentuate the negative?) to shift depression toward enthusiasm. Maybe a new city, or a new specialty, will really be fun. This sounds like some kind of a psychological trick, but in fact the change-meisters claim that every significant change brings about "cognitive restructuring"—i.e., looking at the world differently. So you might as well do it voluntarily.

   Changing the way we feel is hard, because we can't control our autonomic nervous systems; voluntarily changing what we do and what we habitually think about is easier.

5. **Jump out in front of trends and actively get ready for changes.** That will feel a lot better than just being passively reactive, angry, and depressed. Consider making your personal professional goal something that will help you adjust successfully to the changes which are coming your way. If you're working on becoming a computer expert, every time they announce a new operating system or clinical support software, you'll feel you're part of the new world, and on the cutting edge, instead of cut out.

   One physician told me she keeps a private file in her desk labeled "Next." Into this file she stuffs job offers, business cards of contacts in other groups where she might work, and articles on new trends and professional opportunities that she finds interesting. So far she hasn't had to use her Next file, but simply leafing through it occasionally is enough to reassure her that unexpected change won't find her completely unwilling or unprepared.

We docs can no longer afford routinely to be the last to accept every change; we'll just get left farther and farther behind. Our own unwillingness as individual practitioners and as a profession to deal realistically with the inevitable changes in economics, technology, and demographics is contributing to our present problems and creating future ones. Think back twenty years: What if some doc had dug in and said, "Nope, I'm just not going to use computerized scans. I don't like computerization." That doc would be history. At the turn of the last century, many practitioners were pessimistic about all the changes in medicine. They need not have worried: This century turned out to be the greatest medicine has ever seen—so far. Let's not make the mistake they made. The best is definitely yet ahead.

The new gospel: "Blessed are the flexible, for they shall not get their necks broken."

### The Pain of Change

Maybe it won't break our necks, but it would be a lie to say that change is painless. A few years ago I personally agonized through first downsizing and then closing a 150-bed facility. I spent a lot of time staring out my office window, stunned and depressed by the sudden and unavoidable changes and losses.

But within about a year I was able to adjust completely (what other choice did I have?), I was working well with a new team in a new setting—and I had discovered that life goes on after even the biggest disruptions in our professional lives.

However, I do wish that when things were at their blackest, someone had just said to me: "Yes, this is painful. But it will pass.

You're a decent doc, and you're going to be fine on the other side of this."

If you're facing some major upheavals, take that reassurance as being meant for you. If you need to, write it on a card and carry it with you, and read it often. In fact, as I write this, our team is in the rumor stage of another major change, so I'll be following my own advice very soon.

### Why Renoir Kept Painting

The poet Darshan Singh, himself a great artist, often told this story about Pierre Auguste Renoir, whose paintings are so beautiful that each canvas now commands tens of millions of dollars:

When Renoir became older, he developed severe arthritis in his hands and fingers. The pain was so excruciating that he could hardly hold a brush, and every time he painted he suffered physical anguish. Yet in spite of the severe pain it caused him, he would not give up painting. He went on creating masterpiece after masterpiece, holding the brush in his crippled hands as long as he could stand to, enduring tremendous suffering.

Finally a friend of the painter couldn't take it any more. "Renoir, why do you do it?" he implored. "Why do you keep painting, when it obviously causes you such terrible pain?"

Renoir's answer: "My friend, I keep painting because the pain is temporary...but the beauty is forever."

*The pain is temporary, but the beauty is forever.* Let us take the great artist's credo as our own. Right now many physicians are passing through a period of stress and pain. We need to keep in mind that all the previous upheavals of our end-of-millennium century—war, depression, nuclear fear, etc.—have passed. So, inevitably, will this one. Our pain is temporary.

But what you give your patients every day—a return to health, to function, to their families—that is a priceless gift. That is forever.

 **Exercise 17–1** Circle the suggestions below that you will try in your own practice. Add your own suggestions to the end of the list. Keep this book in your office and refer back to this list when you have a moment. Analyze which suggestions are working best for you, and consider whether some others on the list may be worth trying.

1. Get trained in interviewing skills.
2. While interviewing patients, create or continue the relationship.
3. Monitor the problem.
4. Inform, educate, and enlist.
5. Close the encounter.
6. Focus fully on the visit.
7. No unreasonable interruptions.
8. Keep full attention on your patient; make eye contact.
9. Sit close; touch, if appropriate.
10. Allow a brief unstructured moment.
11. Always say something positive and praiseful.
12. Use psychosocial talk.
13. Avoid unprofessional remarks.
14. Speed up, but slow down.

15. Train staff to listen to patients' stories.
16. Get honest feedback about how you come across to patients.
17. Analyze your interaction with patients.
18. Inform your patient constantly about what, why, what next, etc.
19. Share decision making about available treatments.
20. Share actual responsibility for treatment.
21. Give your staff more opportunity to help you.
22. Analyze your role in creating misunderstandings or friction.
23. Remember staff are on your side.
24. Ask staff how they prefer to be addressed.
25. Start a conversation with your staff about whether you are arrogant, etc.
26. Stay alert to how powerfully your words and actions affect co-workers.
27. Set a prestige example.
28. Think about your audience.
29. Include everyone.
30. Woo 'em.
31. Give credit when it's due.
32. Give credit when it's not due.
33. No public bawling out.
34. Get the best people and hold onto them...
35. ...Until you have to let go.
36. Sponsor your staff at educational activities.
37. Have your staff cross-train each other.
38. Show interest in how they do their jobs.
39. Have your staff get efficiency training.
40. Work helpfully with less skilled colleagues.
41. Give unpromising colleagues the benefit of the doubt.

42. Look for the best in a colleague you're quarreling with.
43. Talk it through with her.
44. Realize you're both going for the same goal.
45. Be the first to forgive and forget.
46. Listen to your own body, mind, and spirit.
47. Do something every day to prevent stress buildup.
48. Don't try to hide from change.
49. Hang out with young people.
50. See change as opportunity.
51. Actively prepare for inevitable changes.

(add your own ideas here)

_____

_____

_____

# ✦ 18 ✦

# Afterword: "Have Two Horses"

It has been 100 years since the last popular (it went into 12 printings) self-help book for physicians. Daniel Webster Catthell's *The Book on the Physician Himself and Things That Concern His Reputation and Success* appeared around the time when x-rays, EKGs, aseptic surgery, and internships were transforming medicine into what it became later in the 20th century. The busy practitioners of 1898 needed practical advice on how to proceed into the new era. Among other things, Catthell told them: "Have two horses and drive them singly...that one may be resting, while the other is working."[1(p.21)]

Now you and I are the docs headed into a new century, and again our profession is going through a disorienting transformation. No one can say for sure what the 21st century will bring, but if we could, it probably would seem as exotic and new as the vanished world of "have two horses" seems quaint and outdated. All of us can use help in dealing with the changes we're encountering. This book has tried to be a practical guide to some possible ways to improve and streamline your work.

## No Magic Bullet

If you were looking for a short program—"The One-Minute Doc"—that you could use to give your practice an instant makeover, you may feel disappointed. But as a physician you know the power of methodically attending to details in a complex case, of making small, incremental changes, of going step by step, until you begin to see results. So the approach here has been methodical, incremental, and gradual—not abrupt.

Taken by itself, any one of the 140 suggestions in this book is not earthshaking. However, if you have actually tried putting a few of these ideas to work in your daily practice, and stuck with them, and later tried a few more, then gradually but definitely you have seen a change for the better. In fact—and this is true for all sources of information—what's in these pages is much less important than what you yourself choose to do with it.

## Attitude Matters

If this book has not helped you change anything else, I sincerely wish that you have at least changed your old attitudes. As we've seen, we picked up some of our thought patterns when we were students and residents; they made sense at the time, and first impressions tend to stick. But if these ways of thinking no longer serve us well when we're in practice, we need to replace them.

The first step in changing our attitudes has been to become conscious that we have them, so we can decide whether they fit our present situation. Do you still want other people to set your goals for you? Manage your schedule for you? Tell you what you need to learn and how to learn it? Lead your teams for you? Tell your profession what it ought to be doing and where it ought to be going?

I'm sure you don't want anyone dictating any of these things for you. You are a mature practitioner, not a novice or an apprentice, and only by self-managing your professional life will you attain maximum productivity and satisfaction from your work.

## Changing Hearts and Minds—Starting with Your Own

"Now I understand!" one Beverly Hills specialist exclaimed after a productivity seminar. "This has all been about changing the way I *think!*"

True. It is all about changing the way you think, because how you view the world and how you function in it from moment to moment depend on how your mind works.

But changing your thinking means changing yourself, not other people; and that can be hard to do (just ask a psychiatry resident). Once you've got the hang of it, though, it will give you genuine power over your work, your relationships, and your future.

Gradually, as you begin to take control of this ultimate tool, you find that your whole experience of medical practice starts to change. You're no longer going to work day after day, pushing, rushing, reacting, just getting through it until you can get home to collapse, stunned and exhausted, in front of the TV.

Instead, you move through your day aware that you are each moment choosing, helping, teaching, improving, enjoying, changing the world for the better, one person at a time. Your practice becomes less a hassle and more a labor of love. Each morning you come in smiling at your people and ready for your work, and later you walk out into the evening air and breathe deep and feel good about a job well done.

## What to Do Next

I would suggest that you now put this book away for a few months or a year. Come back to it after you've had time to hang out for a while with the ideas, reflect about your unique practice patterns, and try some of the suggestions. The next time you pick it up, you may get a surprise: Some suggestions that sounded strange on first reading may have become new habits, and some of your old attitudes about practice may already have changed.

> "How many a man has dated a new era in his life from the reading of a book!"
>
> Henry David Thoreau

This book has offered you over 140 ideas for moving in the direction of a more efficient and productive practice, and you'll have hundreds of better ones yourself. Keep thinking for yourself, start putting your good ideas to work in your practice tomorrow, and things will gradually get better for you...and for everyone. Because if physicians become more efficient, that does not mean we're more efficient at making money or producing gadgets. It means we are more efficient and effective at helping more of our patients and their families—and that is a high and worthwhile goal.

> "Derive happiness in oneself from a good day's work."
>
> Henri Matisse[2(p.xxvi)]

Work itself has taste, texture, sweetness—if you take the opportunity to enjoy it, and don't just bolt it. Medicine is the chocolate cake of the professions, and washed down with a little milk of kindness and camaraderie, it can taste very good indeed. I hope you will take every opportunity to enjoy your just desserts.

## And a Few Last Hints

If you've started using some of the suggestions in this book, and have noticed changes for the better in your practice, you may want to consider these final ideas:

1. In order to speed up the learning process, **buddy up with another physician** to discuss and try out more suggestions.

2. Be sure to **fill your new free time with useful activities** that are of a high priority to you personally. You're a doc, so you like to keep occupied.

3. **Don't rub it in with colleagues** if you're now getting things done faster and more smoothly than they are. Instead, do them a favor: Give them a copy of this book, or have the Physician Productivity Seminar at your place, and they can start catching up. If you have found this information useful, they will, also.

4. If you've become good at managing yourself, you may want to **extend your skills to managing others** (on the other hand, you may not). Have you considered becoming chair of your department? Chief of your medical staff? Physician executive? None of us wants to lose that crucial contact with patients, but if each of us serves even a term or two, the administrative work gets done. (That's the line they used when they drafted me to run for chief of staff.)

5. Your three tools are now your servants instead of your masters, but to maintain mastery you'll need to **keep examining your schedule, your knowledge base, your relationships, and your attitudes; never stop changing for the better.**

Finally: Although we've necessarily concentrated in this book on practicing medicine, we also need to keep our larger life in perspective. We were human beings before we became physicians, and after we finish our careers, we will still be humans. Children, spouse, family, friends, community, and our own spiritual work are also parts of being truly human. As we become more efficient physicians, we surely will want to direct more effort into those areas.

Meanwhile, my friend, in your lifelong quest to serve others, I wish you success—and in every working hour, Godspeed.

---

### Notes

1. D.W. Catthell, *The Book on the Physician Himself and Things That Concern His Reputation and Success,* 10th ed. (Philadelphia, PA: F.A. Davis, 1900), 21.
2. H. Matisse, *Jazz* (New York, NY: George Braziller, Inc., 1992), xxvi.

# Index

# 30-Day, Risk-Free Reply Card

# NOTES

# NOTES

# NOTES

# NOTES

# NOTES

# NOTES

# NOTES

# NOTES

# NOTES

# NOTES

# NOTES

# NOTES